FINDING THE EVIDENCE FOR PRACTICE

A Workbook for Health Professionals

Alison Brettle BA(Hons) MSc

Health Care Practice Research and Development Unit, University of Salford, Salford, UK

Maria J. Grant BA(Hons) MSc(Econ)

Salford Centre for Nursing, Midwifery and Collaborative Research,
University of Salford, Salford, UK

Foreword by

Andrew Booth BA MSc DipLib ALA

Senior Lecturer in Evidence Based Healthcare Inf_____ ___nation
Resources, School of Health & Related Research, _____, UK

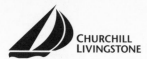

CHURCHILL
LIVINGSTONE

EDINBURGH LONDON NEW YORK OXFORD PHILADELPHIA ST LOUIS SYDNEY TORONTO 2004

CHURCHILL LIVINGSTONE
An imprint of Elsevier Limited

First published 2004

ISBN 0 443 07450 X

British Library Cataloguing in Publication Data
A catalogue record for this book is available from the British Library

Library of Congress Cataloging in Publication Data
A catalog record for this book is available from the Library of Congress

Notice
Medical knowledge is constantly changing. Standard safety precautions must be followed, but as new research and clinical experience broaden our knowledge, changes in treatment and drug therapy may become necessary or appropriate. Readers are advised to check the most current product information provided by the manufacturer of each drug to be administered to verify the recommended dose, the method and duration of administration, and contraindications. It is the responsibility of the practitioner, relying on experience and knowledge of the patient, to determine dosages and the best treatment for each individual patient. Neither the Publisher nor the authors assume any liability for any injury and/or damage to persons or property arising from this publication.
    The URLs quoted were correct at the time of going to press, however, information on the Internet, including URLs, is subject to constant change.

The Publisher

The
Publisher's
policy is to use
**paper manufactured
from sustainable forests**

Printed in China

FINDING THE EVIDENCE FOR PRACTICE

For Churchill Livingstone:

Publishing Director, Health Professions: Mary Law
Project Development Manager: Mairi McCubbin
Project Manager: Samantha Ross
Designer: Judith Wright
Illustrations Manager: Bruce Hogarth

Contents

Foreword   vii

Preface   x

Acknowledgements   xiii

How to use this book   1

| Section 1 | SOURCES OF INFORMATION   5 |

1. Where do I go for information?   7
2. Evidence based sources of information   16
3. The Internet   25

| Section 2 | UNDERTAKING A LITERATURE SEARCH   41 |

4. Approaching the search   43
5. Stages of a search   56
6. Conclusions and final tips   70

| Section 3 | PRACTICAL EXERCISES   79 |

7. Practical exercises   81
8. MEDLINE: Ovid interface   83
9. MEDLINE: SilverPlatter interface (WebSPIRS or WinSPIRS)   96
10. CINAHL: Ovid interface   109
11. CINAHL: SilverPlatter interface (WebSPIRS or WinSPIRS)   122
12. Searching the Internet for healthcare information   135
13. Searching the National Electronic Library for Health (NeLH)   147

| APPENDICES   157 |

Appendix 1 Evaluation tools   159
Appendix 2 Optimal search strategies   165
Appendix 3 Critical appraisal of web sites   167

Glossary   169

Index   173

Foreword

Writing just over a decade after the first appearance of 'evidence based practice' it is difficult to do full justice to the impact this has had on information skills training. Prior to this, literature searching was an activity primarily conducted by librarians and other intermediaries on behalf of their users. Information professionals were just starting to divest themselves of some of the mystique surrounding their practice. Technologically, too, while CD-ROMs opened up the prospect of searching by end users, without the heavy financial penalties of online services, they fell far short of the almost universal access now afforded by the Internet.

The intervening 10 years have seen the appearance of a plethora of books on evidence-based practice including a handful of 'workbooks'. Although the topic of finding the evidence has consistently and rightfully commanded a place as a chapter in such texts, my already sagging bookshelves of evidence-based practice output have yet to identify a workbook specifically on finding the evidence. This then <u>is</u> that book. The authors, Alison Brettle and Maria Grant, are supremely qualified to produce such a book. Reasons for this bold assertion are many, but it will suffice to focus on just three.

With a shared pedigree in health services research both at the internationally renowned *Nuffield Institute for Health* in Leeds and, latterly at the *Health Care Practice Research and Development Unit* and the *Salford Centre for Nursing, Midwifery and Collaborative Research* at the University of Salford, Alison and Maria have been exposed to a wide range of information needs from a demanding and exacting audience. This has undoubtedly shaped their approach both to their own searching practice and to how they communicate this knowledge to others. This legacy is attested to in the extensive involvement of staff and researchers from these units in steering this book as detailed in the Acknowledgements.

Second, both Maria and Alison have enjoyed extensive involvement in conducting literature searching in support of systematic reviews. The technical virtuosity that such intensive activity requires has yielded significant dividends for units such as theirs at Salford and, indeed, my own here at Sheffield. The confidence and competence engendered by searching topics across a wide range of sources and formats has done much to equip a new generation of approachable and accessible 'super searchers', who are able to explain their craft in a way that is easy to understand and to implement.

Lastly, and, arguably, most importantly, Maria and Alison have both established a recent reputation for critically examining the evidence base for their own practice. Whether this is seen in formal interrogation of research evidence relating to information retrieval or other aspects of information practice or, more generally, in an informal questioning of current practice and a quest for continuous improvement, the benefits of such reflective practice for a book like this are clear – practitioners who 'model what they teach' carry credibility and authority.

Of course none of the above provides a compelling reason why you should <u>want</u> to read this book, although, undoubtedly, it should impress on you why you <u>need</u> to do so. For the former I shall turn instead to the ability of both the authors to communicate their knowledge, verbally and in print, with an enthusiasm and exuberance that is infectious. As I read the galley proofs of this book I frequently found myself wanting to try out their exercises in front of my own computer. Indeed, I often wished that I was present to enjoy face-to-face interaction with these two able trainers as they deliver one of their many information skills courses to health service staff. For those of you unable to witness the authors in action, this book provides an extremely satisfying second best.

The three sections of this book are self-sufficient yet complementary. As the authors intend, they can readily be dipped into or systematically explored. While not completely replacing the valued input of a face-to-face training event, they do serve a function analogous to a DIY manual for those unable, or unwilling, to attend the 'evening class'. Perhaps their greatest value, however, lies in their role in consolidating prior learning – for those who have undergone training, but find themselves seeking to recapture or refresh their skills weeks, or even months, after such an event, welcome assistance is at hand.

As you embark on a lifelong pursuit of finding the evidence, to the benefit of patient care and effective organisational practice, I commend this book, to you. If you are a novice before reading this book, you will find your knowledge satisfyingly expanded and broadened. If you are already competent in finding the evidence, you will find reassurance in the tools and techniques outlined and their practical applications. Even information skills 'black belts' will find stimulation for their own practice and for communicating this to others. In your ongoing quest for evidence you will probably find that this concise and well-arranged book is one of the most important sources you encounter.

Advocates of evidence-based practice frequently rehearse the Confucian tenet: 'Give a man a fish you feed him for one day, teach him to fish and you feed him for life'. From the piscatorially improbable locale of Salford, Northern England, the authors deliver a master class in 'netting the evidence' – don't let it be the one that got away!

Andrew Booth

In recent years, access to information has reached unprecedented levels due to the explosion of the Internet. Within healthcare easy access to electronic databases such as MEDLINE has revolutionised the availability of information for teaching, research and practice. Traditionally health professionals have relied on medical libraries or local resources to find information relevant to their practice. However, the current emphasis on evidence based practice and clinical governance, coupled with easier access to electronic information, has shifted the balance, and it is likely that you (as a health professional) have found that you need to carry out a literature search to inform your own practice. Indeed current competencies set out by the NHS Information Authority (2001) require that the majority of health professionals are able to search electronic databases and the Internet in order to meet the targets set out in the NHS Plan (NHS Executive 2001).

Finding relevant information can be frustrating. In theory technology should make finding information easier. However, in reality you may have often found too much information, or nothing relevant to your topic area. You may have found information by accident rather than by design or stopped searching once you had found something vaguely relevant, even if it was not the most appropriate reference. As well as the time involved, this has obvious implications for evidence based practice. A poorly performed search is unlikely to find the best evidence on which to base your practice.

Based on over 10 years experience of teaching health professionals facing these problems, this workbook has been designed with the aim of helping you find information for practice more easily and effectively. General textbooks that cover the theory of literature searching already exist. This one is different. It is highly practical, covers a range of sources and is geared specifically towards health professionals. It does not offer a quick fix – a thorough literature search can (and should) take a long time. However, it will make your searching more systematic and provide you with the opportunities to practise that will increase your confidence in searching. This will in turn improve your ability to locate relevant information for your practice.

Literature searching skills are generic. Once you have mastered some basic techniques, familiarised yourself with the sources of interest to you, and know where to go for help, literature searching becomes easier. Practice helps to reinforce these skills. This workbook is therefore arranged in three sections covering these issues. Each chapter is self-contained, but follows a logical format. You can work through the chapters in turn, or dip into them as required. In our experience, after attending a training session, users often report that they feel confident about searching. However, when they try to do some searching a few weeks or months later, they have forgotten the basic techniques learned. The workbook can be used to remind you of the techniques you learned in a training session. It is also full of practical exercises and tasks that tutors can use or adapt for use in their own training sessions.

The first section covers sources of information and enables you to become familiar with different sources of health information and when it is best to use them. Healthcare information can be found in a wide range of sources. Some are specifically aimed at doctors, some at other professionals and some sources are aimed at a broad range. One of the keys to finding health information is knowing where to look. The first chapter is an introduction to general and health related sources. This is followed by a chapter that focuses on evidence based sources of information. These are often a first port of call for professionals needing to locate quality assured summaries on a particular topic. The final chapter in this section focuses on the Internet, introducing its basic and more advanced search features and how to make the best use of it.

The second section presents a step-by-step guide (or framework) to finding information. It shows you how to clarify what you are looking for and introduces some basic search techniques, primarily relating to electronic database searching, because this is where a large amount of health information can be found. However, once mastered, the majority of these techniques can be transferred to any source.

Finally there is a practical section. Two widely available databases are introduced (MEDLINE and CINAHL) and used to guide you through the process of building up a search strategy in a systematic way. Although MEDLINE and CINAHL are commonly available databases, organisations often access them using different software interfaces. Therefore the exercises are presented for two common interfaces, Ovid and SilverPlatter. There are also practical sections on finding healthcare information via the Internet and the National Electronic Library for Health – a virtual library aimed at providing evidence based information to UK health professionals.

Literature searching is an essential skill for all health professionals, whether you are a trainee or an experienced practitioner. Therefore the book is not aimed at any particular level. It aims to provide something for all levels of knowledge. It gives novice searchers the basic skills to begin literature searching, whilst for those with some literature searching experience, it seeks to challenge common assumptions to literature searching and highlights how these assumptions can impact on the effectiveness of a search.

Throughout the text there are lots of practical examples, tasks and quizzes. These aim to maintain your interest and allow you to check your learning. Where possible we have tried to make these general and relevant to all health professionals. Invariably some examples will not be completely relevant to you. However, it is the techniques you are trying to learn. To a large extent the subject is not important (although we agree that it is more interesting to learn if it is relevant!). Therefore, at the end of each practical, there is a chance to go back and repeat the search on a topic of interest to you.

This book is based on our experiences of teaching literature searching. We have found that all health professionals commonly experience the same frustrations when undertaking literature searching, whether as trainees or once qualified and in practice. The key to improving your searching is confidence and lots of practice. At the end of our workshops users report feeling more confident about their ability to carry out a literature search, and find the evidence they need for practice. Hopefully as a user of the workbook you will shortly feel the same too.

Salford, 2004   *Alison Brettle & Maria J. Grant*

References

NHS Executive 2001 Building the information core: implementing the NHS plan. NHS Executive, Leeds

NHS Information Authority 2001 Health informatics competency profiles for the NHS. NHS Information Authority, Birmingham

Acknowledgements

This workbook has been based on our teaching experiences. However, without the support of a number of people and organisations, it would not have been published for a wider audience. The authors would therefore like to acknowledge their input and support.

The core stakeholder organisations of the Health Care Practice R&D Unit funded the workbook in its original form and staff from these organisations attended our training courses and tested the workbook. These organisations include Bolton Hospitals NHS Trust, Oldham NHS Trust, Rochdale Healthcare NHS Trust, Royal Manchester Children's Hospital, Salford Royal Hospitals NHS Trust, Salford Primary Care Trust and the University of Salford.

The following individuals were involved in reviewing the draft versions of this workbook, and in testing the practical sections. We would like to thank them for their helpful comments. They are: David Brettle, St James' University Hospital, Leeds; Gillian Crofts, Lecturer, Department of Radiography, University of Salford; Holly Day, Health Care Practice R&D Unit, University of Salford; Claire Hulme, Health Care Practice R&D Unit, University of Salford; Sarah Jervis, St James' University Hospital, Leeds; Rosie Kneafsey, Health Care Practice R&D Unit, University of Salford; Andrew F. Long, Health Care Practice R&D Unit, University of Salford; Pat Spoor, Health Sciences Library, University of Leeds; Richard Stephens, Department of Psychology, University of Keele.

We would specifically like to thank Anna Higson, Health Care Practice R&D Unit, University of Salford, for her suggestions and imagination in coordinating the formatting and layout design of the original workbook.

Finally we would like to thank David Brettle, Andrew Long and Richard Stephens for constant support and encouragement.

How to use this book

Evidence based practice involves systematically finding, appraising and using research evidence as the basis for clinical decision-making. It is essential that health professionals aiming to base practice on best evidence gain relevant skills to help find and appraise research evidence. This is a practical guide to gaining some of those skills – those involved in locating information (or finding research evidence). On completing this workbook readers will be more confident in knowing where and how to find evidence (or information).

The workbook uses a practical, case study approach to introduce you to different sources and explain how to use them. The techniques involved are relevant to all sources of information and types of literature searches. Chapter 2 covers sources particularly relevant to evidence based practice.

AIM

The aim of the workbook is to:

- ❏ increase awareness of sources of available information
- ❏ explain the techniques involved in undertaking a literature search
- ❏ demystify some of the jargon associated with computer based literature searching and the Internet
- ❏ help carry out searches efficiently and effectively
- ❏ help practise literature searching techniques.

AUDIENCE

The workbook is suitable for health professionals with very little searching experience as well as those with some searching skills. It could also be used by librarians responsible for training. It was originally produced to be used in conjunction with training sessions provided by the Health Care Practice Research and Development Unit (University of Salford), but it can be used as a stand-alone tool. If used as a stand-alone tool, a basic familiarity with computers (using a mouse and windows interface) is essential.

FORMAT

The workbook is split into three major sections:

- ❏ sources of information
- ❏ undertaking a literature search
- ❏ practical exercises.

The first two sections contain explanations interspersed with tasks to reinforce learning points. At the end of each chapter key points are presented together with a quiz to enable you to monitor your progress. Answers to tasks are also provided at the end of each chapter. The third section comprises practical exercises on searching common health resources. These include MEDLINE and CINAHL (databases frequently used by health professionals), the Internet and the National Electronic Library for Health (NeLH). Suggested answers and guidance on how to find them are provided for the practical exercises.

The workbook provides a general overview of sources. Each local library or information unit may provide some or all of these resources. It is essential to find out what is available to you locally. Your librarian will also be able to help explain some of the techniques and concepts and advise on specialist resources available to you.

EXAMINING YOUR CURRENT PRACTICE

Before you start using this workbook, we would like to examine some of your current search activity and behaviour in relation to literature searching. The aim of this task is to allow you to clarify your current attitudes and approaches to searching for information. At the end of Section 2 we will ask you to examine your attitudes again. Hopefully this will demonstrate a change in your understanding of the tools and techniques you can use, so that future searches will be more efficient and effective.

It is important to remember that there are no right or wrong answers.

Introductory task ATTITUDES TO SEARCHING

Think of ways to describe your approach to literature searching.
For example:

'I just sat down at the computer and did the search . . .'
'I usually just search MEDLINE . . .'
'I only use the Internet . . .'
'I don't bother searching, I just ask a colleague . . .'
'Every time I search I get loads of irrelevant references . . .'
'I know my field and nothing has been published in this area . . .'

What other examples can you think of?

The chapters which follow give you an insight into how some of these statements may shape the type of information you retrieve, and provide tips and techniques on how to search more effectively.

SOURCES OF INFORMATION

1. Where do I go for information?   7
2. Evidence based sources of information   16
3. The Internet   25

CHAPTER 1

Where do I go for information?

AIM

The aim of this section is to introduce you to the range of information sources and their advantages and disadvantages. By the end of the section you should be familiar with the types of resources available and when to use them.

SOURCES OF HEALTHCARE INFORMATION

There is a wide range of different sources of healthcare information available, each with its own advantages and disadvantages and some more suitable to specific needs than others. When looking for information for practice or a research project it is usually necessary to use a range of sources to ensure that a number of angles have been covered (reduce bias). The library is often a key starting point as this provides access to a variety of sources and librarians have the knowledge to point you in the right direction. For those who have access to NHSnet or the Internet, the National Electronic Library for Health (NeLH, http://www.nelh.nhs.uk) is a useful starting point. It provides access to an increasing range of information, particularly evidence based resources.

Once you have found information on the topic of interest, it is necessary to read the information critically (critical appraisal), to ensure the information is of good quality. Some sources, particularly those listed in Chapter 2, are already critically appraised.

Task 1.1 SOURCES OF INFORMATION

Imagine you have been asked to be a member of a working party in your hospital Trust. The working party is to be responsible for developing evidence based guidelines on the management of pain in arthritis. Where would you go for information? List the sources of information you may use. What are the advantages and disadvantages of using them?

Source	Advantage	Disadvantage
1	1	1
2	2	2
3	3	3
4	4	4

Below are some of the sources you may have listed – together with their advantages and disadvantages. Note: They are listed in alphabetical order, not order of preference or suggested use.

Books

A first stage in many literature searches, books can be comprehensive, pulling together a wide range of perspectives. On the downside they may be out of date as it can take a long time for books to be written, edited and published. New editions of classic texts are published regularly.

Colleagues

Colleagues are a useful source of information. They are easily accessible and may provide you with a relevant answer quickly or point you towards another useful source of information. However, when carrying out research or looking for information based on evidence, colleagues may not be the most accurate or up-to-date point of reference.

Electronic databases and indexes

Databases and indexes can be used to track down journal articles and other types of information such as conferences and reports. There are many available in healthcare and related fields, ranging from large internationally focused databases such as the American biomedical database MEDLINE, to smaller locally developed databases such as those produced for internal use by organisations. Table 1 lists a selection of these.

Table 1 Selected health related databases

Database	Description	Availability
AMED – Allied and Alternative Medicine	Produced by the British Library Health Care Information Service. Covers physiotherapy, occupational therapy, rehabilitation, podiatry and complementary medicine from 1985. Printed format is Physiotherapy Index, OT Index etc	CD-ROM, online
ASSIA – Applied Social Science Index	Covers all aspects of the social sciences including community care and social aspects of health and welfare. Printed version available	CD-ROM, online
British Nursing Index (BNI)	Covers popular and important journals in nursing and midwifery. Focuses on mainly British journals	CD-ROM, NeLH (to UK NHS staff), online
CINAHL – Cumulative Index to Nursing and Allied Health Literature	Covers nursing and allied health disciplines, including physiotherapy and health education from 1983 onwards. Strong US focus	CD-ROM, NeLH (to UK NHS staff), online

table continues

Database	Description	Availability
Cochrane Library	Specialised database giving access to a range of systematic reviews carried out by the Cochrane Collaboration and the NHS Centre for Reviews and Dissemination. Also contains register of randomised controlled trials	CD-ROM in medical and health libraries NeLH (to UK NHS staff), online
CSP Databases	Databases of physiotherapy research in progress/recently completed and database of physiotherapy specific documents	Via Chartered Society of Physiotherapists
DH-Data	Health service and hospital administration with a focus on the UK NHS, toxicology and environmental health. Contains full text of many Department of Health documents	NeLH (to UK NHS staff), online
Embase	Biomedical literature from 110 countries with a strong coverage of European material, particularly in relation to drugs and toxicology; 3500 journals are indexed from 1974 onwards. Printed version is Excerpta Medica	CD-ROM, NeLH (to UK NHS staff), online
MEDLINE	General biomedical database produced by the National Library of Medicine in the USA. Covers international literature on medicine including allied health, biological and physical sciences and humanities. From 1966 to present. Covers 3700 journals worldwide. The printed version is Index Medicus	CD-ROM, NeLH (to UK NHS staff)
PsycInfo (Psychlit)	Produced by the American Psychological Association. Covers psychology, treatment and prevention, social and educational psychology, clinical and behavioural studies	CD-ROM, NeLH (to UK NHS staff), online
Sociofile	Covers sociology	CD-ROM, online

Indexes are paper based lists of references to articles that can be searched by subject or author, but as these are slow and unwieldy to use, they have largely been replaced by computerised databases.

A database is a collection of information held on computer. Often this is statistical data or contact details, but databases have become widely used to track down journal articles or relevant information. Databases are provided on CD-ROM or online via a host computer. You may need to go to a library to access them. Each database covers a slightly different topic area. If your topic of interest covers a range of perspectives, it will be necessary to search a range of databases. Some are available free of charge via the Internet; others can be accessed for a fee or may have been made available via your library.

Databases are made up of records usually comprising the reference for the article, an abstract (summary of the article) and keywords (describing the content of the article). The allocation of keywords is known as indexing. Because of the way these records are indexed retrieving the information you want is not always easy. Common problems are retrieving too much information or retrieving lots of irrelevant information. The techniques described in Chapters 4 and 5 aim to overcome these problems.

Internet

A source of information that has recently received a lot of media publicity is the Internet. This connects thousands of computer networks, linking up millions of computers, and provides easy, fast communication for a vast number of computer and network users throughout the world. The Internet is not one source of information – but a way of accessing many kinds of sources – a global electronic library. The Internet contains masses of information on all kinds of topics, some of it useful, but unfortunately much of it not. It is difficult to know whether a site is authoritative or not and it can be difficult to find what you want amongst the mass of available information. Information can be published very quickly and often it is relatively easy to obtain usually obscure information via the Internet. The Internet is covered in much greater detail in Chapter 3.

Journals

Journals are likely to provide more up-to-date information than books but there is still sometimes a publishing delay. There are many journals available, but they can be difficult to access and it can be difficult to keep up-to-date with what has been published. Some hospital departments may have their own journal collections or you may have to obtain articles via a library or inter-library loan.

Professional organisations

Professional organisations provide a wide range of services, including publications, and in some cases have their own specialist information services and/or databases that are available to members. There are many different organisations. Professionals are often aware of organisations that are relevant to them; others can be tracked down via directories or the Internet.

Reports

Reports are produced regularly by government departments, Royal Colleges, academic organisations and other statutory and voluntary organisations. Reports often cover a particular topic area aimed at a limited readership. They can be a source of information that is not published in any other form, drawing together a range of perspectives. They sometimes cover new and rapidly developing technologies, summarising the state of the evidence. They are often difficult to track down. Report literature is sometimes called 'grey' or 'unpublished' literature.

Hopefully you are now more familiar with different sources of information available and their limitations. Because of the nature of sources, some are more appropriate than others for particular tasks. This does not mean that other sources will not lead you to the information you want – but selecting one source over another may be more efficient.

KEY POINTS

❏ There is a wide range of sources available.

❏ Different sources have different coverage.

❏ In the course of a literature search it is often important to use a variety of sources to ensure comprehensiveness and reduce bias.

❏ Even with a good knowledge of sources and access to the Internet, the library is still an essential place to visit when undertaking a literature search of any kind. The librarian will usually have a good knowledge of the subject area and how to access specific resources.

? QUIZ

a) Which are the most appropriate sources when locating the following types of information?

Type of information   **Most appropriate source**

1. Background information or trying to get a
   feel for a topic?

2. Current information on a particular topic?

3. Journal articles on a particular topic area?

4. A particular journal reference?

5. A book reference or the books available on
   a topic?

6. Reports published by a particular organisation
   and perhaps obtain a copy of it?

7. A copy of a journal article?

8. Recently published information or an
   obscure topic?

b) Why is it important
   to use a range of
   sources?

SUGGESTED ANSWERS

Task 1.1: Suggested answers

Imagine you have been asked to be a member of a working party in your hospital Trust. The working party is to be responsible for developing evidence based guidelines on the management of pain in arthritis. Where would you go for information? List the sources of information you may use. What are the advantages and disadvantages of using them?

Information for guidelines can be obtained from any of the sources mentioned in this section. However the following are probably the most useful.

Source	Advantage	Disadvantage
Electronic databases	They will lead you to the wide range of **journal articles** publishing the most up-to-date evidence. Specific databases may include MEDLINE, Embase and the Cochrane Library	May find too much information. May not have relevant journal articles available locally. May not have most appropriate databases locally
The Internet	There are a number of sites providing information on guidelines via the Internet. Internet searches may also lead you to relevant reports published by **professional organisations**	The quality of some of the sites may be questionable. Need to find a way through the mass of irrelevant information
Professional organisations	Organisations such as the British Rheumatological Society, Arthritis Research Campaign or Chartered Society of Physiotherapists may have produced some guidelines, a **report** or carried out some research in this area	This type of information can be scattered and difficult to track down

Quiz: Suggested answers

a) Which are the most appropriate sources when locating the following types of information?

Type of information	Most appropriate source

1. Background information or trying to get a feel for a topic? → Books / Reports

2. Current information on a particular topic? → Journal articles

3. Journal articles on a particular topic area? → Electronic database / Index

4. A particular journal reference? → Electronic database

5. A book reference or the books available on a topic? → Local library

6. Reports published by a particular organisation and perhaps obtain a copy of it? → The organisation / The Internet / Local library

7. A copy of a journal article? → Local library / Inter-library loan / The Internet (possibly)

8. Recently published information or an obscure topic? → The Internet

b) Why is it important to use a range of sources? → It is essential to use a range of sources of information to reduce bias (ensure all angles of the argument/research have been covered) and ensure comprehensiveness.

Evidence based sources of information

This chapter aims to provide an insight into the range of evidence based information sources and the diverse ways in which evidence based information can be presented. Many of the resources listed below are available via the Internet. However, you will be encouraged to visit your library and information service to find out what resources are available to you locally.

 EVIDENCE BASED SOURCES OF INFORMATION

In Chapter 1 you were introduced to the range of general information sources you might use in meeting your information needs, and were encouraged to consider when you might most appropriately use these sources of information. You will now be given an insight into the diverse range of evidence based sources within these groups.

Two of the main advantages of evidence based sources of information is that their quality is often evaluated for you and they can, in many instances, provide a review of up-to-date evidence available for a particular topic area. There is a range of evaluation tools you can use, and courses or journal clubs you can attend, to develop a thorough understanding of critical appraisal. (See Appendix 1.)

Clinical effectiveness literature can be obtained from a wide range of publications, databases and organisations. The guide which follows aims to provide an indicative first point of call.

The Internet, which is often viewed as an important resource in its own right, provides access to a range of information sources, some evaluated, some not. The majority of resources listed below are available via the Internet, and an opportunity will be provided to search many of these web sites in the practical exercises in Section 3. If you are unfamiliar with searching the Internet, please read Chapter 3 before attempting to access any of the web sites. Details of how to search for and evaluate alternative sources of information on the Internet are also included in Chapter 3.

Journals and newsletters

Journals and newsletters can be useful to obtain up-to-date information on research evidence. From general clinical information to specialist subjects, the number and range of evidence based publications have dramatically increased in recent years, ranging from in-house publications, to internationally peer reviewed journals. Electronic databases can provide a useful way of keeping abreast of research evidence published beyond those journals you have easy access to. (See pages 9–11 for further details.)

A variety of journal and newsletter formats are available from academic to newsy or digest approaches.

Bandolier (www.jr2.ox.ac.uk/bandolier) adopts an informal brief approach to the presentation of its information, but cites the evidence for its recommendations. Its target audience is healthcare commissioners, to assist them in keeping up-to-date with local and national initiatives on the effectiveness of healthcare interventions.

A more formal approach is adopted in the subject-specific journals *Evidence Based Medicine, Evidence Based Midwifery, Evidence Based Mental Health* and *Evidence Based Nursing*. These journals are published with specific sectors of the healthcare professions in mind, and provide detailed abstracts and commentaries from published studies and reviews in order to keep health service professionals up-to-date with important advances in treatment, prevention, diagnosis, cause, prognosis and the economics of internal medicine.

Digests form an important part of the journal and newsletter literature, providing a short summary of research evidence which is referenced to enable you to follow up any areas of particular interest. Examples include the bi-monthly bulletin *Effective Health Care (EHC)* (www.york.ac.uk/inst/crd/ehcb.htm), which is based on systematic reviews and synthesis of research evidence; *Effectiveness Matters* (www.york.ac.uk/inst/crd/em.htm), which complements EHC and provides updates on the effectiveness of interventions; and *Health Evidence Bulletins* (http://hebw.uwcm.ac.uk) as produced by the Welsh Office.

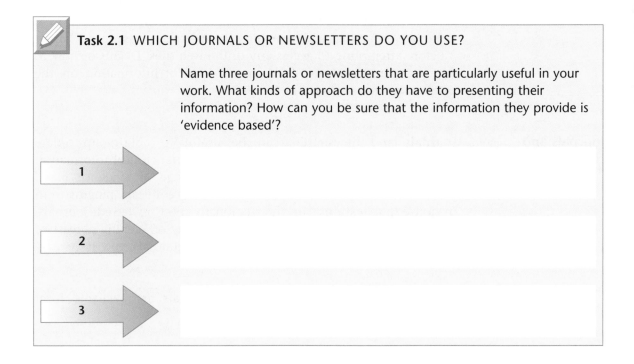

Task 2.1 WHICH JOURNALS OR NEWSLETTERS DO YOU USE?

Name three journals or newsletters that are particularly useful in your work. What kinds of approach do they have to presenting their information? How can you be sure that the information they provide is 'evidence based'?

1

2

3

Organisations

Professional and charitable organisations and associations can be an important source of grey literature. Below are some examples of national organisations specialising in evidence based information.

The *Cochrane Collaboration* is an international network of individuals working to prepare, maintain and disseminate systematic and up-to-date reviews of healthcare effects. The collaboration produces 'The Cochrane Library', a well-known database of systematic review evidence. Web site: www.cochrane.de

The *Irish Clearing House on Health Outcomes (ICHHO)* acts as a focal point for networking and supporting the exchange of ideas and practice experience in relation to health outcomes. Future developments include the development of a web site providing access to UK and European sources of information on outcomes, health indicators and evidence based practice. Web site: www.ich.ie/ichouse

As the largest independent social research and development charity in the UK, the *Joseph Rowntree Foundation* supports a wide programme of research and development in the areas of housing, social care and disability, young people and families, and work, income and social policy. The Foundation is a good source of report literature. Web site: www.jrf.org.uk

NHS Centre for Reviews and Dissemination (CRD) in York seeks to provide services to promote awareness and access to quality reviews of research evidence. Web site: www.york.ac.uk/inst/crd/welcome.htm

The *National Institute for Clinical Excellence (NICE)* works with clinical bodies to systematically appraise health interventions before they are introduced into the National Health Service and produce advice and guidelines. Web site: www.nice.org.uk

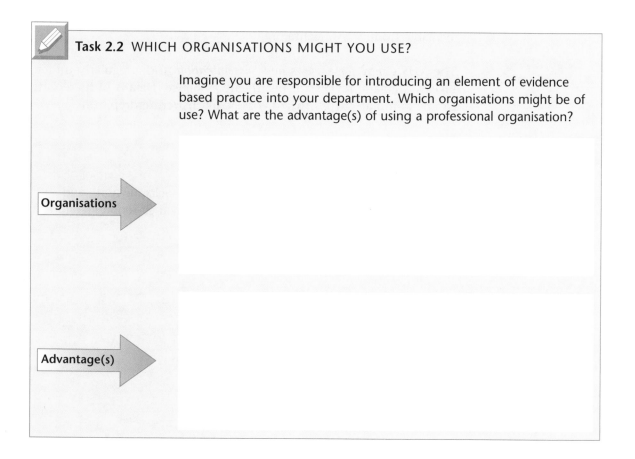

Task 2.2 WHICH ORGANISATIONS MIGHT YOU USE?

Imagine you are responsible for introducing an element of evidence based practice into your department. Which organisations might be of use? What are the advantage(s) of using a professional organisation?

Organisations

Advantage(s)

Reports

Often referred to as 'grey literature', reports can provide a useful means of drawing together information from a range of perspectives.

Reports are regularly produced by government departments, Royal Colleges, universities and voluntary and self-help groups. It is not possible to list all potentially relevant report producers here. The organisations described below specialise in providing evidence based reports at a national level.

The *Aggressive Research Intelligence Facility (ARIF)* seeks to help health-care workers by providing access to and advice on existing reviews of research evidence. Web site: www.bham.ac.uk/arif/

The *National Coordinating Centre for Health Technology Assessment (NCCHTA)* is responsible for the Department of Health's HTA programme. The purpose of the programme is to ensure that high quality research information on the costs, effectiveness and broader impact of health technologies is produced in the most effective way for those who use, manage and provide care in the NHS. Its reports are available from: www.ncchta.org/

The *NHS Centre for Reviews and Dissemination (CRD)* regularly undertakes systematic reviews of healthcare evidence. Details of its reports can be found at: http://nhscrd.york.ac.uk/inst/crd/crdrep.htm

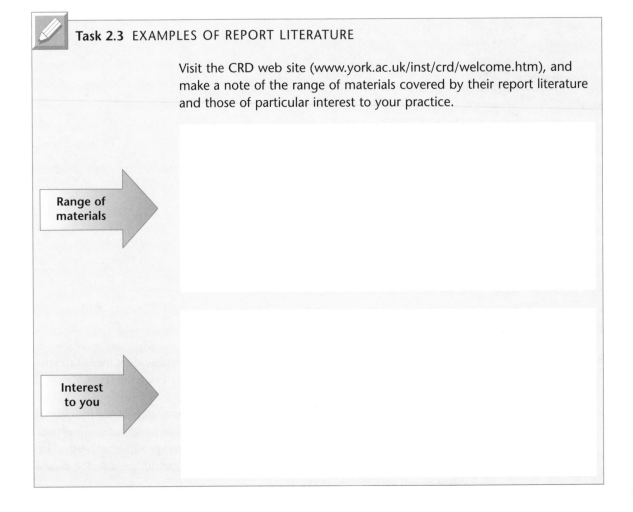

Task 2.3 EXAMPLES OF REPORT LITERATURE

Visit the CRD web site (www.york.ac.uk/inst/crd/welcome.htm), and make a note of the range of materials covered by their report literature and those of particular interest to your practice.

Range of materials

Interest to you

Databases

In addition to the general bibliographic databases listed in Chapter 1 (see pages 9–11), some databases are particularly useful when searching for evidence based information as they provide commentaries or reviews of the information they contain.

Best Evidence brings together the abstracts and commentaries of the evidence based journals *ACP Journal Club and Evidence Based Medicine* with the full text of *Diagnostic Strategies for Common Medical Problems.* It includes: structured abstracts; expert commentary putting the information into a clinical perspective; best diagnostic tests and strategies; the benefits and harms of interventions; and questions commonly raised by practising physicians. Further information is available from: www.bmjpg.com/

The *Cochrane Library* is a regularly updated electronic library that facilitates access to a range of databases. These include: The *Cochrane Database of Systematic Reviews (CDSR),* a rapidly growing collection of regularly updated systematic reviews of the effects of healthcare; the *Database of Abstracts of Reviews of Effects (DARE),* which provides structured abstracts of published systematic reviews; the *Cochrane Central Register of (CENTRAL) Controlled Trials Register (CCTR),* a bibliography of over 100 000 controlled trials; and the *Cochrane Methodology Register (CMR),* a bibliography of articles on the science of research synthesis and on practical aspects of preparing systematic reviews. The Cochrane Library is available via the National Electronic Library for Health (NeLH). Web site: www.nelh.nhs.uk

The *TRIP Database* searches across 58 sites of high-quality medical information, providing hyperlinked access to evidence based material on the web as well as articles from online journals such as the *British Medical Journal* (BMJ), the *Journal of the American Medical Association* (JAMA), and the *New England Journal of Medicine* (NEJM). Web site: www.tripdatabase.com

These databases provide a good first step in locating summaries or reviews of the literature in particular topic areas. However, where they do not meet your information needs, you will need to search more widely (using the sources listed in Chapter 1, and the search techniques outlined in Section 2). Some organisations have produced search strategies (sometimes referred to as search filters or optimal search strategies) to assist in you in identifying specific types of research more effectively. Examples of some of these search strategies can be found in Appendix 2.

Task 2.4 DATABASE AVAILABILITY AND COVERAGE

Visit your local library and information service, and find out which databases are available to search. What topic areas do they cover?

KEY POINTS

❑ There is a diverse range of evidence based resources available.

❑ Evidence based sources comprise critically appraised information – often in summary form.

❑ Evidence based resources provide a good starting point.

❑ For topic areas that are not covered, it is necessary to use the general resources outlined in Chapter 1.

? QUIZ

1. What are the advantages of using evidence based sources of information?

2. How can you be sure that information is evidence based?

SUGGESTED ANSWERS

Task 2.1: Suggested answers

Name three journals or newsletters that are particularly useful in your work. What kinds of approach do they have to presenting their information? How can you be sure that the information they provide is 'evidence based'?

There are a number of ways of assessing whether information presented in journals and newsletters is likely to be of good quality or is evidence based.

One indicator of possible quality is if a publication is peer reviewed. You can normally identify peer reviewed journals from the guidance to authors notes. If it is peer reviewed, then the information presented will have been through a process whereby experts in the field will have scrutinised and commented upon its contents prior to publication. A publication can seem to be of good quality even if it is not peer reviewed. One way to assess this is to check if the information presented is supported by references to other resources, and then critically appraise its contents yourself!

Task 2.2: Suggested answers

Imagine you are responsible for introducing an element of evidence based practice into your department. Which organisations might be of use? What are the advantage(s) of using a professional organisation?

Organisations
NHS Centre for Reviews and Dissemination – produces high quality systematic reviews on a range of topics.
National Institute of Clinical Excellence (NICE) – produces guidance and guidelines on a growing number of topic areas.
Any professional organisation related to your subject area/specialism.

Advantage(s)
Organisations/professional bodies often produce or commission reports that bring together information from a range of perspectives, summarising the evidence.

Task 2.3: Suggested answers

Visit the CRD web site (www.york.ac.uk/inst/crd/welcome.htm), and make a note of the range of materials covered by their report literature and those of particular interest to your practice.

The NHS Centre for Reviews and Dissemination has produced a range of report literature, providing an in-depth discussion of the results of systematic reviews undertaken, including those produced as part of the *Effective Health Care Bulletin* series.

Quiz: Suggested answers

1. What advantages are there from using evidence based sources of information?

Evidence based sources of information are often evaluated and can provide reviews of up-to-date evidence in particular topic areas.

2. How can you be sure that information is evidence based?

Evidence based sources of information provide references to resources in support of any statements made and provide details of how they are compiled.

The Internet

The aim of this chapter is to introduce you to the Internet, its jargon and some of its potential uses. You will also learn about some of the Internet based services you can use to find information more efficiently.

 THE INTERNET

The rapid development of the Internet in recent years has made it a popular first choice for people searching for information. However, there is often some confusion about what constitutes the Internet. A good definition comes from the *Evidence Based Social Care Newsletter*. It states:

> [the Internet is] an international 'network of networks' of computers linked together ... [which enable you] to have the ability to communicate with others anywhere in the world (ESBC 1999)

From this definition it is clear that the Internet provides a means of accessing information and resources in a variety of forms. For example, information may be provided as a web page or via a web page to a searchable database, e.g. MEDLINE.

The Internet can provide access to information on all kinds of topics, of varying quality and usefulness. Technological developments mean it is possible for anyone to put information on the Internet, and it can be difficult to know whether a site is authoritative or not. However, by using some of the tools and techniques listed below, and by critically appraising the information, you can have increased confidence in the quality of the information you access.

TERMINOLOGY

You may have come across lots of jargon in relation to the Internet. Task 3.1 aims to improve your knowledge of Internet related terminology.

Task 3.1 TERMINOLOGY

See if you can match up the terms with the definitions.

Applets	A hierarchical and structured database of information that provides a means of searching the Internet
Browser	The storage of copies of web pages previously retrieved so that the speed of future retrievals is enhanced. To ensure that the most current information is presented, the program compares the date of the stored copy with the file at the original location
Caching	The sending of text files (in the form of messages) to be sent from one computer to another
Directory	Self-contained programs that can be incorporated into web pages
Email	A facility for moving files between computers on the Internet
FTP (File Transfer Protocol)	The process of linking one web page to another
Gateway service	A program used to view web pages, e.g. Internet Explorer or Netscape Navigator
Hypertext links	Provides access to selected sites in a particular subject area
Internet	Operate by creating a locally indexed database of web pages as a means of searching the World Wide Web

Java Script or JScript	Free service to enable discussion of issues and sharing of information *via a bulletin board*
Mailing lists	A condensed file which enables large documents to be stored and sent quickly and easily
Newsgroups	Provides access to value added services such as directories and sites providing links to related web sites
PDF (Portable Document File)	A programming language that can be used to enhance the interactivity of web pages
Portal	The publishing side of the Internet, which allows files placed on the web to be accessed
Search engine	An international 'network of networks' of computers linked together
Vortal	Free serice to enable discussion of issues and sharing of information *via email*
WWW (World Wide Web)	Provides access to value added services such as directories for specific user groups, perhaps defined by subject areas

The range of terms used in relation to the Internet is huge, but this list provides you with a good overview of some of the most frequently used, and will help you as you proceed through the rest of this chapter.

Web browser

A web browser is a program used to view web pages. Internet Explorer and Netscape Navigator are two of the most common web browsers used. Both adopt a similar way of presenting information. Let's take a closer look (Figure 3.1).

Figure 3.1 Health Care Practice Research and Development Unit web page. Reproduced with permission.

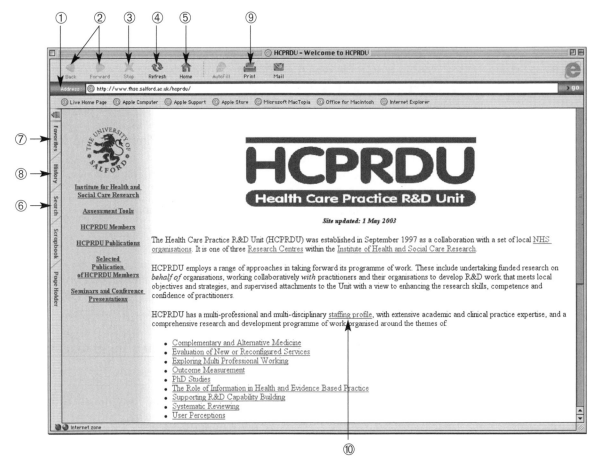

① The *'address bar'* is sometimes referred to as the *'location bar'* or the *'URL'* (Uniform Resource Locator). This is the place where you type a web page address, pressing the *'return button'* or *'enter button'* on your keyboard to load the web page. Web addresses usually begin with http:// e.g. http://www.fhsc.salford.ac.uk/hcprdu/ (see below). By clicking on the downward arrow at the end of the address bar, you should see a list of the web addresses you have typed in.

② The *'back and forward buttons'* allow you to return to web pages you have previously visited during the session. Currently shaded out on this web browser, the *'forward button'* becomes activated once you have used the *'back button'*.

③ The *'stop button'* allows you to stop loading a web page. For example, you may wish to stop loading a page if it is taking too long to appear in your web browser.

④ The *'refresh button'* allows you to reload the page currently displayed in your web browser. You may wish to do this to update the 'cached' or stored version of the page on your computer. For example, you may wish to reload the BBC News web page to check on the most current news story.

⑤ The *'home button'* allows you to return to the web page originally loaded when you opened your web browser.

⑥ The *'search button'* will take you to the preferred search engine of the web browser you have loaded on your computer. You can then undertake a search of World Wide Web. More details on how to get the most from you search engine appear later in this chapter.

⑦ The *'favourites button'* is sometimes referred to as the *'bookmark'*. The feature allows you to store the addresses of web pages you have found useful and may wish to revisit at a later date.

Your list of favourites can be organised in a similar way to the file manager you use to organise your word documents.

⑧ The *'history button'* allows you to review the list of web pages you have visited within a set period of time, e.g. today, yesterday, last week etc.

⑨ The *'print button'* allows you to print the current web page displayed on your web browser.

⑩ Most web pages include *'hypertext links'* to enable you to visit other web pages. The text of hypertext links is usually blue and underlined, although sometimes a hypertext link is hidden or 'embedded' within a picture. You can tell if an image or piece of text is a hypertext link because your mouse icon will change from an arrow to a hand as it moves over it. Click on the hypertext link to visit the next web page.

Find function

There is one other feature on your web browser that you may find useful. At the top of the web browser there is a menu of functions similar to those on your word processing package, e.g. 'file', 'edit', 'view', 'favourites', 'tools' and 'help'. By clicking on the 'edit' menu, you will see an option to 'Find (on this page)'. This will allow you to search for a word or phrase on the web page you currently have loaded on your web browser, and it can be a very useful feature if the page is very long!

How is the web site address composed?

Web site addresses each follow the same structure, including a protocol, a site address, and a location of a resource within that site. Web site addresses are case sensitive, so they must be entered into the address bar ① carefully or the web site may not be found. An example of a web site address is:

http://www.fhsc.salford.ac.uk/hcprdu/events.htm

Protocol   Site address   Location of resource within site

The 'Protocol' tells the computer how to access the web page. Most pages can be accessed using http, which stands for hypertext transfer protocol. The http protocol is an industry standard, and is so common most web addresses no longer include it when citing their web address. For example, the web site address for the *British Medical Journal* (BMJ) is simply: www.bmj.com

Web pages are loaded onto computers or servers, and the 'Site address' tells your computer where it needs to search on the Internet to find a particular computer or server. The above web address indicates that the web page is loaded at www.fhsc.salford.ac.uk a web server of the University of Salford.

Within web sites there are often numerous subpages or resources, which are separated in the web site address by a '/'. In the web site address for the Health Care Practice Research and Development Unit above, we can see that there are two levels of resources within this web site. The 'events' resource is part of the 'hcprdu' resource, which is a part of the www.fhsc.salford.ac.uk web site. It is common for web resources to move, but for web sites to remain. Therefore if you have problems accessing a particular web resource it is sometimes useful to reduce the web address to a previous '/'. For example:

www.fhsc.salford.ac.uk/hcprdu/events.html

If this web page does not load, remove the last-named web resource to the previous '/':

www.fhsc.salford.ac.uk/hcprdu/

And if this resource does not load, remove the last-named web resource, to go back to the main web site address:

www.fhsc.salford.ac.uk/

Task 3.2 USING YOUR WEB BROWSER

Log on to your computer, and open your web browser. Practise typing the following web site addresses into the address bar ①, following hypertext links ⑩ and using the buttons at the top of the web browser to move backward and forward, returning to the home page, reloading pages. Remember to use the help screen if you have any queries or questions about using the browser.

Here are three web site addresses you might like to practise with:

- ❑ British Medical Journal: www.bmj.com/
- ❑ Health Care Practice Research and Development Unit: www.fhsc.salford.ac.uk/hcprdu/
- ❑ NHS Centre for Reviews and Dissemination: www.york.ac.uk/inst/crd/welcome.htm

Notes:

FINDING INFORMATION ON THE INTERNET

Search engines

Search engines enable you to find information on a particular topic via the Internet using a word or phrase. Using software programs called 'spiders', 'robots' or 'crawlers', search engines operate by creating, and then searching, a locally indexed database of web pages. The spiders, robots or crawlers run automatically to check existing pages, and index new resources, so the range of material indexed can be quite diverse.

Each search engine also operates slightly differently, and so you can retrieve quite different results depending on the search engine you use. Research has suggested that, at best, a search engine is likely to have indexed only 34% of the Internet (Lawrence and Giles 1998), so if you do not find what you want first time, try a different engine.

Although using a search engine is similar to searching a database, there are some important differences. For example, when searching a database you can specify the field you wish a word to appear in. So, if you wish to retrieve papers written by Andrew Long, you could restrict your search to finding the occurrence of *Long* in the author field. However, when using a search engine, it would look for any occurrence of the word *Long* anywhere on the web page. Some search engines will also automatically 'default' to a truncation function (described in Chapter 5), and search for any words which begin with the stem of a word, e.g. if you typed in the word *Long*, it would retrieve anything relating to 'long' or 'longed' or 'longing' etc. One technique to help you overcome this when searching the Internet is the use of phrasing. Phrasing means searching for phrases by using quotation marks, e.g. 'Andrew Long'. If words are enclosed in quotation marks, the search engine will retrieve documents in which the words appear together.

Most search engines have a simple and an advanced search feature, which can result in different web sites being retrieved (Figures 3.2 and 3.3). This is because the search features operate in different ways. The main advantage of using the advanced search feature is that you can make your search more precise by controlling the use of some of the techniques, such as truncation and Boolean operators, described in Chapter 5.

When you are using a search engine, the web site details that are retrieved are likely to be ranked in order or relevance. However, what is considered relevant by the search engine may not be what you consider relevant, so check the help screen for details of how the results of your search will be presented.

Figure 3.2 Example of a 'simple' search feature.

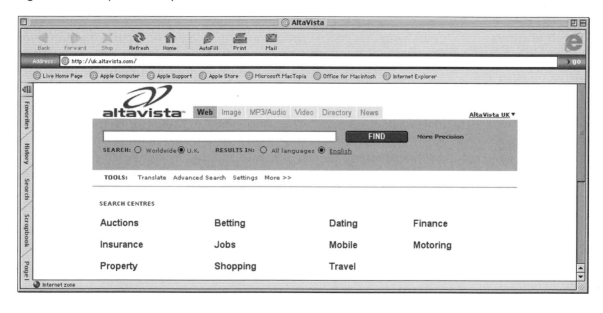

Figure 3.3 Example of an 'advanced' search feature.

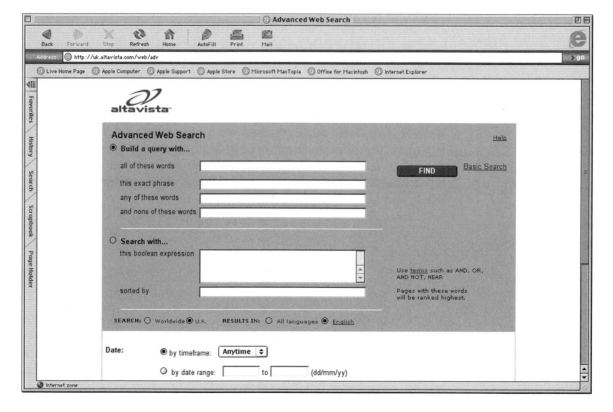

Check the help screen of each new search engine to familiarise yourself with the search commands before you get started. *Do not assume that all search engines use the same search commands.*

Examples of search engines include:

Alta Vista: www.altavista.com
Excite: www.excite.com
Hot Bot: http://hotbot.lycos.com
Lycos: http://lycos.cs.cmu.edu
MSN: www.msn.com

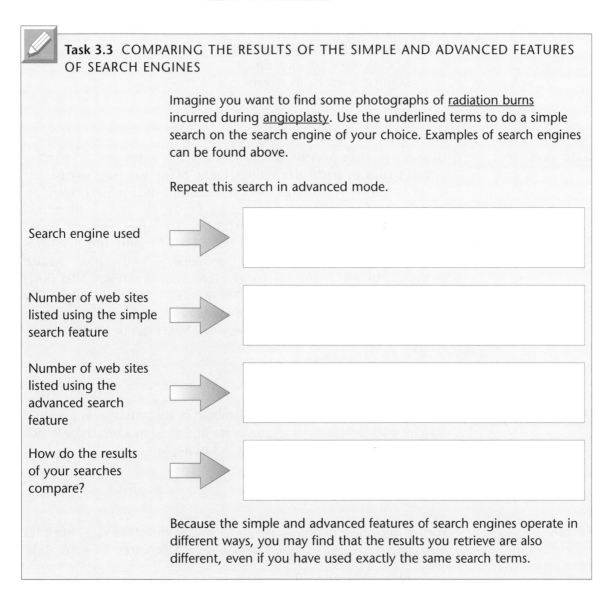

Task 3.3 COMPARING THE RESULTS OF THE SIMPLE AND ADVANCED FEATURES OF SEARCH ENGINES

Imagine you want to find some photographs of <u>radiation burns</u> incurred during <u>angioplasty</u>. Use the underlined terms to do a simple search on the search engine of your choice. Examples of search engines can be found above.

Repeat this search in advanced mode.

Search engine used

Number of web sites listed using the simple search feature

Number of web sites listed using the advanced search feature

How do the results of your searches compare?

Because the simple and advanced features of search engines operate in different ways, you may find that the results you retrieve are also different, even if you have used exactly the same search terms.

Meta search engines

Meta search engines work by searching a range of search engines and presenting the information back in a single list. They aim to overcome some of the problems of coverage by individual search engines. Each meta search engine operates using a different set of search engines. As with individual search engines, you may need to use a range of meta search engines in order to find the information you require. On the downside, although you are likely to retrieve an increased number of relevant sites, you are also likely to retrieve more irrelevant material.

Examples include:

Ask Jeeves: www.ask.co.uk
Copernic: www.copernic.com
Google: www.google.com
Ixquick: www.ixquick.com
MetaCrawler: www.metacrawler.com

Gateways

Gateway services provide access to searchable catalogues of selected Internet sites in particular subject areas. Many gateway services are quality assessed. A list of gateway services and their subject coverages is provided by the University of Leeds at: www.leeds.ac.uk/ ROADS/subject-listing/service/000.2.html Examples include *OMNI* (http://omni.ac.uk), which covers the areas of health and medicine, NMAP, which covers nursing, midwifery and allied health (http://nmap.ac.uk), and the patient information gateway *NHS Direct Online* (www.nhsdirect.nhs.uk). *The National Electronic Library for Health (NeLH)* is also an example of a gateway service, providing access to a wide range of health related services. NeLH can be accessed at:

www.nelh.nhs.uk

Directories

A directory utilises a structured database of information as a way of searching the Internet. Its resources are organised in a hierarchy which allows users to browse its contents. An example is:

Yahoo: www.yahoo.com

Portals

Portals provide an access point to value added services such as directories and sites providing links to related web sites. An example is:

AOL: www.aol.com

Vortals

Vortals are similar to portals in that they facilitate access to value added services such as directories and sites providing links to related web sites. However, unlike portals, vortals are subject specific. An example is:

Netting the Evidence: www.nettingtheevidence.org.uk

APPRAISING INFORMATION

Whilst many rating systems are used on the Internet, it is often unclear on what criteria a web site's accreditation has been achieved. There is no regulatory body monitoring the information available on the Internet. It is therefore important to critically appraise the information you obtain from the Internet.

Critical appraisal helps to ensure that information is of good quality and makes sound, evidence based, recommendations. This is true of all information sources whether presented in a book or a journal paper. Although similar criteria apply to most resources (e.g. credibility of the author, currency etc.), specific checklists have also been designed for appraising information found on the Internet. An example is the 'Quality Information Checklist' (www.quick.org.uk/menu.htm). This provides a set of eight questions, with illustrative examples. (See Appendix 3.)

KEY POINTS

❏ The Internet is a good resource providing access to a wide range of information.

❏ Finding the information you want can be difficult.

❏ Search tools such as directories and gateways are useful for finding topic-specific evaluated resources efficiently.

❏ Search engines and meta search engines are an alternative means of finding information.

❏ The quality of the information on the Internet can be variable. Information retrieved should always be critically appraised.

? QUIZ

1. Why should you critically appraise web sites before using the information they present?

2. If you cannot find the information you seek using a search engine, what alternative search tools can you use?

SUGGESTED ANSWERS

Task 3.1: Suggested answers

See if you can match up the terms with the definitions

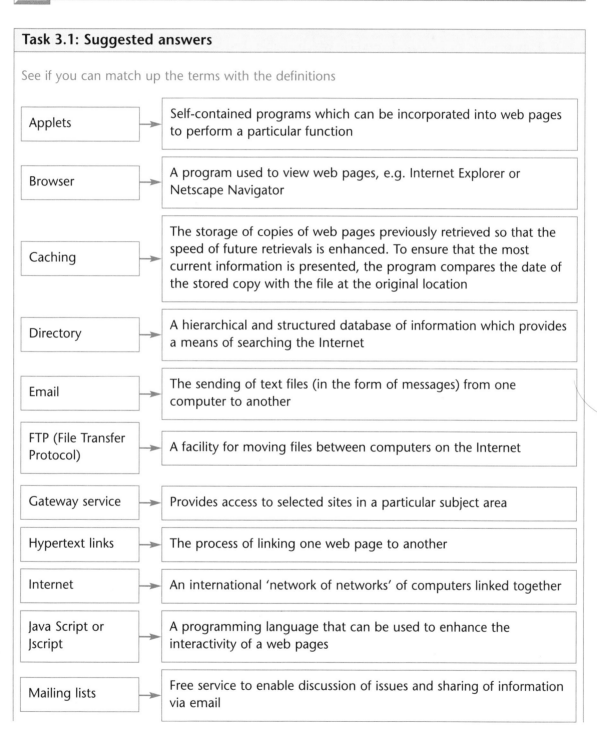

| Applets | → | Self-contained programs which can be incorporated into web pages to perform a particular function |

| Browser | → | A program used to view web pages, e.g. Internet Explorer or Netscape Navigator |

| Caching | → | The storage of copies of web pages previously retrieved so that the speed of future retrievals is enhanced. To ensure that the most current information is presented, the program compares the date of the stored copy with the file at the original location |

| Directory | → | A hierarchical and structured database of information which provides a means of searching the Internet |

| Email | → | The sending of text files (in the form of messages) from one computer to another |

| FTP (File Transfer Protocol) | → | A facility for moving files between computers on the Internet |

| Gateway service | → | Provides access to selected sites in a particular subject area |

| Hypertext links | → | The process of linking one web page to another |

| Internet | → | An international 'network of networks' of computers linked together |

| Java Script or Jscript | → | A programming language that can be used to enhance the interactivity of a web pages |

| Mailing lists | → | Free service to enable discussion of issues and sharing of information via email |

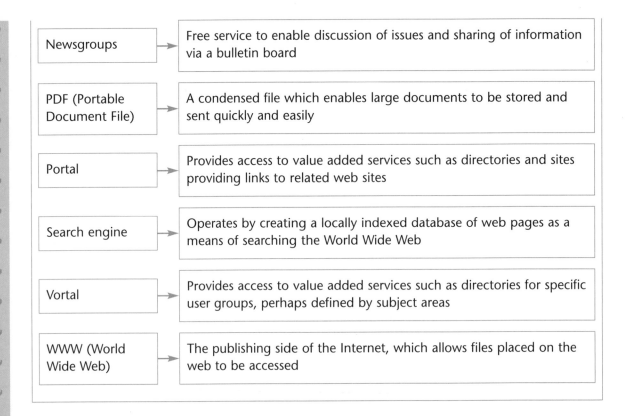

Newsgroups	Free service to enable discussion of issues and sharing of information via a bulletin board
PDF (Portable Document File)	A condensed file which enables large documents to be stored and sent quickly and easily
Portal	Provides access to value added services such as directories and sites providing links to related web sites
Search engine	Operates by creating a locally indexed database of web pages as a means of searching the World Wide Web
Vortal	Provides access to value added services such as directories for specific user groups, perhaps defined by subject areas
WWW (World Wide Web)	The publishing side of the Internet, which allows files placed on the web to be accessed

Task 3.3: Suggested answers

Imagine you want to find some photographs of <u>radiation burns</u> incurred during <u>angioplasty</u>. Use the underlined terms to do a simple search on the search engine of your choice. Examples of search engines can be found on page 33.

Having used the example of finding some photographs of radiation burns incurred during angioplasty, you will have selected two search terms or phrases and undertaken both a simple and advanced search on the search engine of your choice.

You may have found that the results in terms of numbers and sites you retrieved were different, even if you used exactly the same search terms. This is because the simple and advanced features of search engines operate in different ways.

Quiz: Suggested answers

1. Why should you critically appraise web sites before using the information they present?

As with all information sources you should be confident about its quality and evidence base. The quality of web sites is particularly open to ambiguity because of the ease with which new sites can be established. Fortunately several Internet specific checklists exist to enable you to critically appraise information presented on web pages. See Appendix 3 for further details.

2. If you cannot find the information you seek using a search engine, what alternative search tools can you use?

As well as using alternative search tools such as subject gateways or vortals, you could also try using different search engines. Remember, at any one time a search engine is likely to cover a maximum of 34% of Internet based resources.

References

ESBC 1999 Evidence Based Social Care Newsletter, Issue 5, Summer, p2
Lawrence S, Giles C L 1998 Searching the world wide web. Science 3: 98–100

SECTION 2

UNDERTAKING A LITERATURE SEARCH

4. Approaching the search   43

5. Stages of a search   56

6. Conclusions and final tips   70

Approaching the search

Chapters 4–6 outline a systematic approach to a literature search. They also illustrate how to turn your ideas for a topic for research into a search question. Using this type of approach will make your search for information more efficient and effective.

 LITERATURE SEARCHING

A literature search is a search for information using a range of sources. It will usually include published sources of information, but in some cases it will also include grey literature (or unpublished information).

Before beginning a search it is essential to think about the information you want and how you are going to get it – and therefore make your search more efficient. If you are not clear before starting the search, it is easy to get side-tracked by information you find along the way, and waste valuable time and effort. Considering the five questions below will provide a more structured and systematic approach to your search.

1. WHY are you doing the search?

Do you want to find a couple of references to back up some ideas you have for a presentation? Do you have to complete an assignment for a college course? Are you trying to introduce an aspect of evidence based practice into your work? Are you undertaking a literature review for an MSc, PhD or major research project? Are you part of a team undertaking a systematic review? Each scenario requires a different approach to the search.

Finding a couple of references to back up an argument is very different to undertaking a systematic review. For the former, providing you find the information you require, it does not matter what you miss. For a systematic review you need to find all the evidence available – mainly primary research and including published and unpublished sources. If you are introducing an aspect of evidence based practice, you will probably want to find reviews and overviews that have been undertaken by others which summarise the available evidence. In both these cases missing information could have serious implications for the conclusions of the review or on your practice. For a piece of academic work someone else may have already done something similar to your proposed research. Depending on the level of your research, you may be able to build on their approach or you may need to modify your research so as not to duplicate.

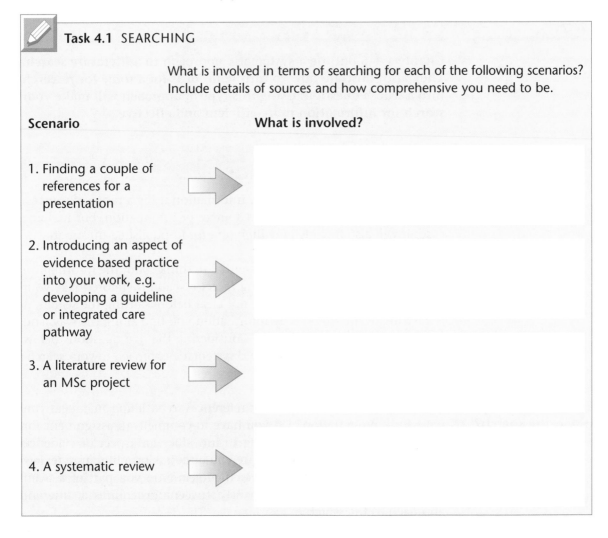

Task 4.1 SEARCHING

What is involved in terms of searching for each of the following scenarios? Include details of sources and how comprehensive you need to be.

Scenario	What is involved?
1. Finding a couple of references for a presentation	
2. Introducing an aspect of evidence based practice into your work, e.g. developing a guideline or integrated care pathway	
3. A literature review for an MSc project	
4. A systematic review	

2. WHAT are you searching for?

What is your research about? What is your search question? Being clear and focused about the topic you are researching makes it easier to undertake a search, deal with the information retrieved and draw more meaningful conclusions. Sometimes you may have little choice about the topic of the search. If you are being commissioned or requested to do a search, you may need to go back to the originator for clarity or with ideas for how to make the search question more focused. Further help on formulating search questions is provided below (pages 46, 49).

3. WHAT are your constraints?

You may be restricted by time or the sources of information you have access to. Depending on WHY you are undertaking the search you may have to find ways round some of these constraints. If you are limited by time or have access to limited resources, you may have to accept that your search will not be as comprehensive as you may have wished.

4. WHAT sources?

What sources are suitable for the topic area? Do you need to search multiple sources? Do you have access to the sources you need to search? Your librarian may be able to give you some advice in answering these questions. Which sources can you realistically search in the time you have available to find the information you need?

5. HOW comprehensive?

How comprehensive does your search need to be? Do you need to find one viewpoint? Do you need to find all the primary research covering all aspects of the topic area? Do you need to identify the main relevant themes?

Think back over the previous questions. When searching you are usually aiming to strike a balance between sensitivity (recall) – the *amount* of available information on your search question – and precision – the proportion of *relevant* information retrieved. These two concepts are inversely correlated. The more comprehensive your search needs to be, the more sensitive (broad) your search should be. This means that you will need to wade through lots of irrelevant references to ensure that you do not miss important ones.

Remember that to be comprehensive it is essential to use a wide range of sources. Different databases have different coverage. Searching multiple databases increases the comprehensiveness but will still miss some material because not all journals are covered or there may be indexing problems. Handsearching journals and using other sources will significantly improve comprehensiveness. However, you also need to consider what is manageable. There is little point in searching a large range of sources if you cannot deal with the information you have retrieved. The aim is to try and strike a balance between how comprehensive you need to be and what you can manage. This is not always easy!

Conclusion

Answering these questions will focus the approach to your search. Writing down your answers to these questions will help to form a search plan. Once involved in a search you can revisit your plan to ensure that you are on the right track or modify your plan in light of the results you obtain from your searching.

THE SEARCH QUESTION

Before beginning a search it is essential to clarify your search question. The key to ensuring that the search is manageable (as well as being realistic about the time involved) is having a clear search question. In other words, think about what you are searching for. This will ultimately make your search for information much easier and will help you to develop your search strategy.

Common problems are:

❏ Vagueness

For example:

→ I'm looking for information on managing pressure sores.
→ Is rehabilitation effective?

These types of questions would result in thousands of references.

❏ Too complicated when dealing with an obscure topic

For example:

→ I'm looking for information on the neuropsychological effects of impacts to the head as experienced by professional footballers in Cardiff.

These types of questions would result in too few references or the searcher possibly being led to believe that nothing has been published on that particular subject.

❏ Too complex – should really be more than one topic

For example:

→ What is multiprofessional working and why does it work?

There are several questions here, the definition of multiprofessional working, the effectiveness of multiprofessional working and the elements of multiprofessional working which may be effective. So the question could be broken down into a number of questions.

Phrasing your topic as a question

One method to help clarify your ideas is to phrase your topic as a question. It may be necessary to include more information in your question such as the population or condition or intervention you are interested in.

For example:

→ I'm looking for information on managing pressure sores

could become:

→ Are pressure-relieving beds/mattresses effective in the management of pressure sores?

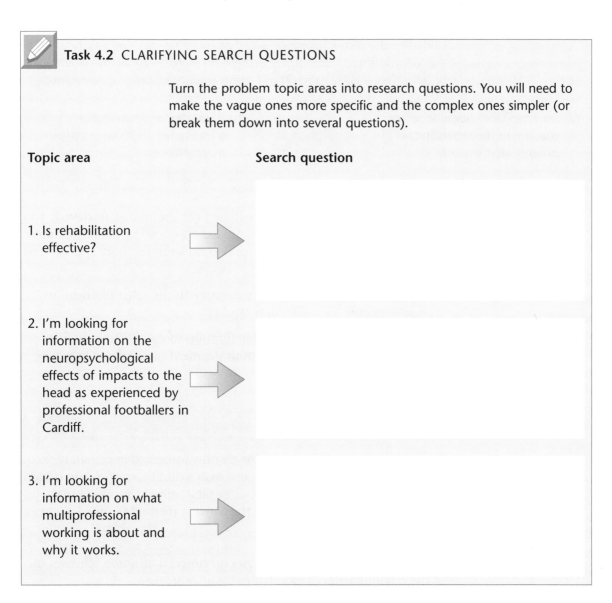

Task 4.2 CLARIFYING SEARCH QUESTIONS

Turn the problem topic areas into research questions. You will need to make the vague ones more specific and the complex ones simpler (or break them down into several questions).

Topic area

Search question

1. Is rehabilitation effective?

2. I'm looking for information on the neuropsychological effects of impacts to the head as experienced by professional footballers in Cardiff.

3. I'm looking for information on what multiprofessional working is about and why it works.

Once you have identified a question from your topic area, you need to break it down into distinct, manageable concepts or components. These concepts will later be used as 'building blocks' in your search strategy. There may be two or more concepts in your search question.

For example:

→ Are <u>pressure relieving beds/mattresses</u> effective in the management of <u>pressure sores</u>?

Task 4.3 IDENTIFYING IMPORTANT CONCEPTS

Underline the distinct components that could be used for searching in the following questions. Tip: Searching on words such as 'management' or 'effective' is likely to result in a large amount of irrelevant references.

(a) Are hospital at home schemes effective in the rehabilitation of patients after stroke?

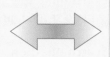

(b) Is vocational rehabilitation effective for adults with severe mental illness?

During the course of the search (based on the results retrieved) you may find you need to modify your search question making it more general or specific. To make the previous examples more specific you could add the concepts underlined below.

→ Are <u>hospital at home schemes</u> effective in the rehabilitation of <u>elderly people</u> (over 65) after <u>stroke</u>?

→ Is <u>payment</u> for <u>vocational rehabilitation</u> more effective than <u>vocational rehabilitation without</u> payment for adults with <u>severe mental illness</u>?

LIMITING SEARCHES

If you get too much information or are only interested in certain types of research methodologies, you may also wish to limit your search to certain types of studies – systematic reviews or randomised controlled trials, for example. This can be done using the concept method outlined above.

For example:

→ Are there any systematic reviews on hospital at home schemes in the rehabilitation of elderly people after stroke?

You may decide to change your question later – depending on the results of an initial search. For example, a search restricted to elderly people or stroke may result in too few studies. Alternatives could be:

→ Are there any <u>systematic reviews</u> on <u>hospital at home schemes</u> for <u>elderly people</u>?
→ Are there any <u>systematic reviews</u> on <u>hospital at home schemes</u> after <u>stroke</u>?

Building up a search on different concepts as demonstrated above allows you to refine your search as you proceed. Some database 'experts' have developed search strategies which identify certain types of studies (e.g. randomised controlled trials or systematic reviews). These can be combined with your subject terms. An example is listed in Appendix 2. Alternatively some database packages have limit features (including publication type, language, publication year, age).

AN ALTERNATIVE METHOD OF FORMULATING A SEARCH QUESTION – PICO

An alternative method of clarifying your search question is the PICO method (University Library, University of Illinois at Chicago 2003). This is based on the principles outlined above, but offers a more structured approach. It involves breaking a topic down into three or four parts and is often suited to very clinical questions.

For example, if you were interested in whether St John's wort was effective when used as an antidepressant, you could break down the question in the following manner:

P – Patient or Problem
   Define the patient or problem being addressed
   e.g. adults with mild depression
I – Intervention
   Define the intervention or treatment being considered
   e.g. St John's wort
C – Comparison
   Give a comparison
   e.g. traditional antidepressants or no treatment
   (NB: This item may not be necessary for some questions)
O – Outcome
   Describe the clinical outcome(s) or outcome of interest
   e.g. reduction in depression

These categories equate to the concepts described in the method above and can be used to build up your search strategy.

Task 4.4 DEVELOPING A SEARCH PLAN

Imagine you are on a committee for developing evidence based guidelines for pain relief in arthritis. Use the five questions to set out a search plan.

Question	Response
1. Why are you doing the search?	
2. What are you searching for? (Use the concept or PICO approach to formulate your search question.)	
3. What are your constraints?	
4. What sources?	
5. How comprehensive?	

KEY POINTS

❏ It is essential to prepare for the literature search before undertaking any actual searching.

❏ Focusing or clarifying your search question is the key to ensuring you do not end up with a mass of irrelevant information.

❏ Thinking about sources and how comprehensive your search needs to be ensures that you do not get side-tracked or miss information.

❏ Using a five question approach leads to efficient and effective searching.

? QUIZ

Question	Response
1. Why should you prepare a search beforehand?	
2. Why does a search when undertaking a systematic review or finding information for evidence based practice need to be comprehensive?	
3. Name a common problem with search questions?	
4. What does PICO stand for?	

SUGGESTED ANSWERS

Task 4.1: Suggested answers

What is involved in terms of searching for each of the following scenarios? Include details of sources and how comprehensive you need to be.

Scenario	What is involved?

Scenario

What is involved?

1. Finding a couple of references for a presentation

A quick database search or ask a colleague.

2. Introducing an aspect of evidence based practice into your work, e.g. developing a guideline or integrated care pathway

Thorough and detailed search using a wide range of sources, particularly those mentioned in the chapter on evidence based practice. May need to seek help from a librarian or information professional. It will be more useful (and quicker) to search for reviews already undertaken rather than searching for primary research evidence.

3. A literature review for an MSc project

A thorough search using a range of sources to provide a balanced review. It is more important to ensure that all arguments are covered than find every relevant paper or study.

4. A systematic review

A thorough and comprehensive search using a wide range of sources, including contacting experts and making efforts to track down unpublished reports. It is essential to locate as many primary research studies as possible and cover all themes and arguments to ensure bias is not introduced into the review conclusions. It is essential to seek the advice of a librarian or information professional.

Task 4.2: Suggested answers

You could have developed any question relating to these topics. Hopefully your answers will be something like those suggested below.

Topic | **Search question**

1. Is rehabilitation effective?

1. Are hospital at home schemes effective in the rehabilitation of patients after stroke?
2. Is vocational rehabilitation effective for adults with severe mental illness?

2. I'm looking for information on the neuropsychological effects of impacts to the head as experienced by professional footballers in Cardiff.

Do footballers experience neuropsychological problems caused by impacts to the head?

3. What is multiprofessional working? Does it work? If so why?

1. What is the definition of multiprofessional working?
2. What is the role of communication in the effectiveness of multiprofessional working?

Task 4.3: Suggested answers

Underline the distinct components that could be used for searching in the following questions.

(a) Are <u>hospital at home schemes</u> effective in the <u>rehabilitation</u> of patients after <u>stroke</u>?

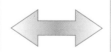

(b) Is <u>vocational rehabilitation</u> effective for <u>adults</u> with <u>severe mental illness</u>?

Task 4.4: Suggested answers

Imagine you are on a committee for developing evidence based guidelines for pain relief in arthritis. Use the five questions to set out a search plan.

Question

Response

1. Why are you doing the search?

→

To introduce an evidence based guideline for arthritis across the trust.

2. What are you searching for? (Use the concept or PICO approach to formulate your search question.)

→

What are effective methods of pain relief for arthritis? NB: This may need to be further split into drug related and non-drug related. To look at all methods in one project is probably too large. What are effective drugs in the treatment of arthritis? What non-pharmacological interventions are effective in treating arthritis?

3. What are your constraints?

→

Three months to undertake project. Staff to undertake project in addition to normal duties. Can only use resources in hospital library.

4. What sources?

→

Cochrane Library, MEDLINE, locally available journals and knowledge of clinicians.

5. How comprehensive?

→

Limit to published systematic reviews. Accept that some reviews may be missed if you have limited access to sources.

Quiz: Suggested answers

Question	Response
1. Why should you prepare a search beforehand?	To reduce the likelihood of missing information, retrieving too much irrelevant information and ensure that your search is effective.
2. Why does a search when undertaking a systematic review or finding information for evidence based practice need to be comprehensive?	To ensure that you reduce bias and you are basing your conclusions on all sides of the argument (as much available evidence as possible relating to the intervention).
3. Name a common problem with search questions?	Vagueness or complexity.
4. What does PICO stand for?	Patient/problem, Intervention, Comparison Outcome – a method of focusing search questions.

Reference

University Library, University of Illinois at Chicago 2003 Evidence Based Medicine. Finding the best clinical literature, formulating patient centred questions. Web site: www.uic.edu/depts/lib/lhsp/resources/pico.shtml

CHAPTER 5

Stages of a search

AIM

This chapter aims to show how you turn your search question into a search strategy. It will also show you techniques you can use to get the information you want rather than a mass of irrelevant references.

 ## STAGES OF SEARCHING

There are six main stages of a search. These are:

1. Clarify your search question (described in Chapter 4, pages 46, 49).
2. Identify the most important components for searching (described in Chapter 4, page 48).
3. Translate your concepts into terms used by the database you are searching.
4. Identify a range of synonyms to describe your concepts.
5. Combine concepts using Boolean operators.
6. Review results and revisit steps 1–5 in light of results.

It is important to note that although these stages appear to happen one after another, in practice literature searching is an iterative spiral rather than a linear process. It may be necessary to revisit each of the stages at various times and modify the approach throughout the search. Searches are rarely perfect first time – even when you have years of searching experience.

The approach and techniques described below are particularly aimed at electronic database searching. However, the principles of searching are the same whether you are using paper based sources, electronic databases or the Internet.

The points made in this chapter should become clearer once you have completed the practical exercises in Section 3. You may wish to reread this section after completing the practical. Alternatively you could read part of this chapter, complete the relevant practical exercise and then go on to the next part of the chapter.

Databases comprise thousands of electronic records. Each record describes a particular item such as an article in a journal or in some cases books or reports. A typical record is shown in Figure 5.1. Each record is divided into fields that contain pieces of information such as authors, source and abstract.

Figure 5.1 An Ovid MEDLINE record. Reprinted with permission of Ovid Technologies, Inc. All rights reserved.

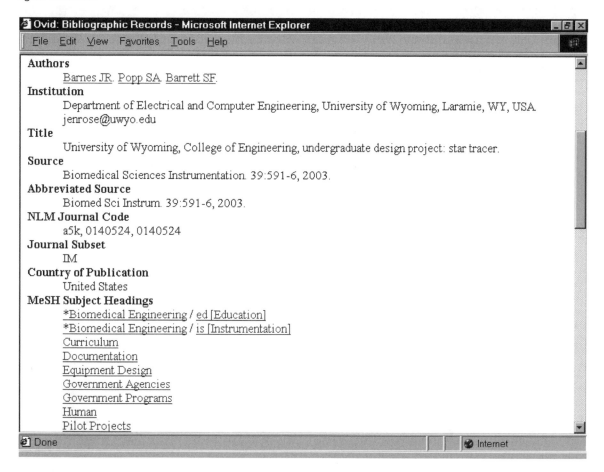

If you are unfamiliar with database searching, you may wish to log on to MEDLINE at this point to familiarise yourself with a database. MEDLINE should be available via your local medical library, perhaps on your hospital network or a free version of MEDLINE is available via the Internet at:

www.ncbi.nlm.nih.gov/PubMed/

In addition to this information, each record is 'indexed' according to its subject by a professional indexer. These 'index' terms are often selected from a 'controlled' list of vocabulary used to describe particular concepts. Index terms are also known as keywords, subject headings, or in the case of MEDLINE, MESH (medical subject headings). They may be structured into a thesaurus or arranged in a hierarchy.

Figure 5.2 MESH hierarchy for the term 'rehabilitation'. Reprinted with permission of Ovid Technologies, Inc. All rights reserved.

An example of part of the MESH hierarchy is shown in Figure 5.2.

Ovid: Tree - Microsoft Internet Explorer					
File Edit View Favorites Tools Help					
☐ Patient Isolation	1694	☐	☐	ⓘ	
+ ☐ Physical Therapy Techniques	16213	☐	☐	ⓘ	
☐ Placebos	23047	☐	☐	ⓘ	
☐ Prescriptions, Non-Drug	749	☐	☐	ⓘ	
+ ☐ Punctures	7878	☐	☐	ⓘ	
+ ☐ Radiotherapy	18610	☐	☐	ⓘ	
− ☑ Rehabilitation	9113	☐	☐	ⓘ	
☐ Activities of Daily Living	24022	☐	☐	ⓘ	
☐ Art Therapy	626	☐	☐	ⓘ	
☐ Bibliotherapy	175	☐	☐	ⓘ	
☐ Dance Therapy	86	☐	☐	ⓘ	
☐ Early Ambulation	1125	☐	☐	ⓘ	
☐ Music Therapy	1004	☐	☐	ⓘ	
☐ Occupational Therapy	5568	☐	☐	ⓘ	
+ ☐ Physical Therapy Techniques	16213	☐	☐	ⓘ	
+ ☐ Rehabilitation of Hearing Impaired	1031	☐	☐	ⓘ	
+ ☐ Rehabilitation of Speech and Language Disorders	0	☐	☐	ⓘ	
☐ Rehabilitation, Vocational	6489	☐	☐	ⓘ	
☐ Rejuvenation	149	☐	☐	ⓘ	
☐ Remission Induction	16228	☐	☐	ⓘ	
+ ☐ Renal Replacement Therapy	1120	☐	☐	ⓘ	
+ ☐ Reproductive Techniques	3657	☐	☐	ⓘ	
+ ☐ Respiratory Therapy	4106	☐	☐	ⓘ	
Done				Internet	
				Tuesday, July 15, 2003	

The hierarchy is arranged from general to specific. Scope notes provide explanations of what is covered by each term. Indexers select the most appropriate specific term to describe the subject in question. Therefore if you are interested in the general topic of rehabilitation you will need to select this and all the narrower terms under it. (Most MEDLINE packages allow you to 'explode' the term so that all the narrower concepts are included in your search.) Searching on index terms (keywords, MESH) is a good method of retrieving the most relevant articles to your subject area. However, in practice you can miss relevant articles or retrieve irrelevant ones as different indexers may choose a different term to describe the concept in question or miss an important subject element of an article.

Stage 3: Translating your concepts into terms used by the database

Once you have clarified the question and broken it down into the important concepts as described in Chapter 4, it is necessary to translate these concepts into terms that will be recognised by the database – the index terms (keywords/MESH). This will ensure that you retrieve the articles that are most relevant to your search question. You will need to identify index terms for each of your important concepts.

Some database packages (including these on the Ovid and SilverPlatter interfaces) allow you to type in a term and then will suggest the most appropriate term to use. Others allow you to search the index. Some database interfaces do not offer this feature and you may need to type in a term and look at the results obtained to see how the relevant records have been indexed. There may be more than one index term

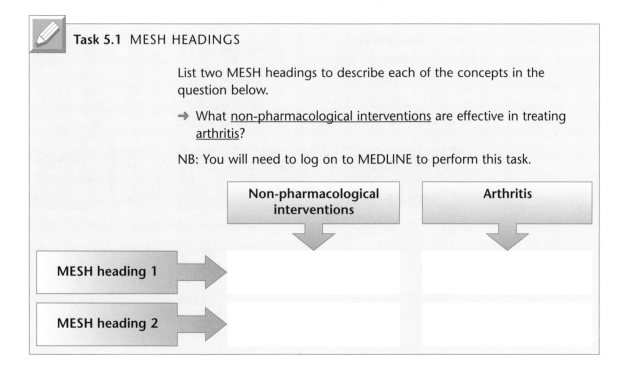

Task 5.1 MESH HEADINGS

List two MESH headings to describe each of the concepts in the question below.

→ What <u>non-pharmacological interventions</u> are effective in treating <u>arthritis</u>?

NB: You will need to log on to MEDLINE to perform this task.

	Non-pharmacological interventions	Arthritis
MESH heading 1		
MESH heading 2		

relevant to your concept and you will need to search on all the relevant terms to obtain the information you need.

Stage 4: Identify synonyms to describe your concepts

To ensure your search is comprehensive, or to search for a concept which is not adequately covered by the index terms or to overcome inadequate indexing, it is necessary to search free text. This is sometimes known as text word searching. This means that you type in your term and search for it, usually in the title and abstract fields.

There is usually a range of words (synonyms) that can be used to describe the concepts in your search question. These need to be included in your search plan and then later in your search strategy in addition to the subject headings you have already found.

For example, in the search question:

→ Are <u>hospital at home schemes</u> effective in the <u>rehabilitation</u> of patients after <u>stroke</u>?

The following synonyms could be used to describe the different concepts:

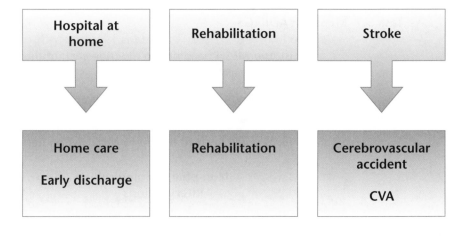

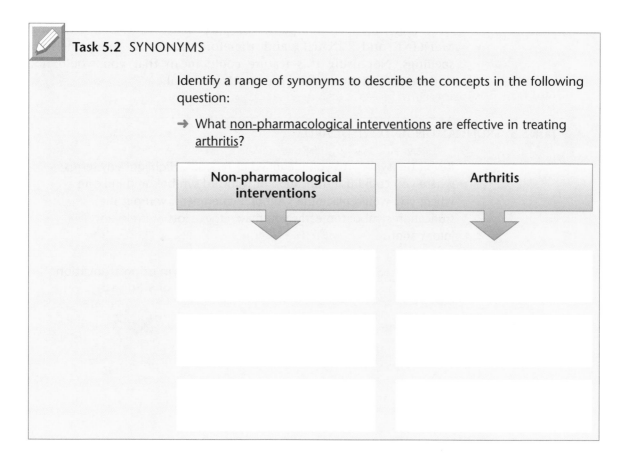

Task 5.2 SYNONYMS

Identify a range of synonyms to describe the concepts in the following question:

→ What <u>non-pharmacological interventions</u> are effective in treating <u>arthritis</u>?

Non-pharmacological interventions	Arthritis

When you type in a term the database will usually look for the word exactly as you have spelled it. To ensure that you search for variations of words, plurals and different spellings the following features are useful.

Truncation

By entering the stem of a word followed by a symbol (usually * or $), all words beginning with that stem will be retrieved. For example:

Manage* will retrieve manage, manager, management etc.

Different software packages use different symbols. Check the help screens to find the truncation symbol for your software package before beginning your search.

Wildcards

This feature replaces one (in some cases more than one) letter and is useful in searching for different spellings. (Usually a ?) For example:

→ Organi?ation would retrieve organisation or organization.

Note that American companies produce many databases, including MEDLINE and CINAHL, and therefore frequently use American spellings. Not using this feature could mean that you would not retrieve a lot of either American or UK material.

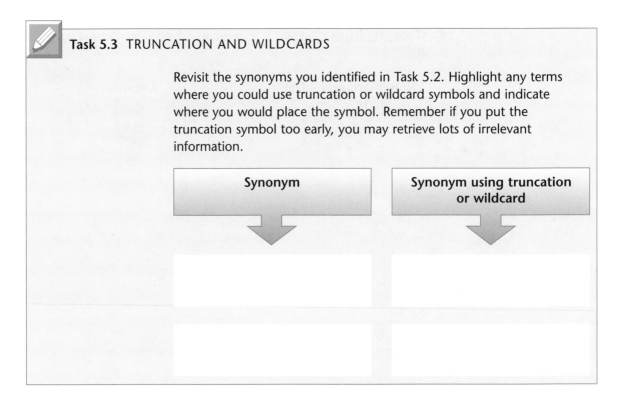

Task 5.3 TRUNCATION AND WILDCARDS

Revisit the synonyms you identified in Task 5.2. Highlight any terms where you could use truncation or wildcard symbols and indicate where you would place the symbol. Remember if you put the truncation symbol too early, you may retrieve lots of irrelevant information.

Synonym	Synonym using truncation or wildcard

If your search does not need to be particularly comprehensive, you may be able to miss out this stage.

Stage 5: Combine concepts using Boolean operators

You now have a range of ways of describing your search question. To ensure that you retrieve relevant references, you need to combine all these terms together. To combine these different concepts in a search you will use Boolean operators. These are logical operators that enable you to broaden or restrict a search. The main operators are 'OR' and 'AND'. These allow you to combine the terms for each of your concepts and then combine them with each other.

The following Venn diagrams illustrate how they are used.

The OR operator

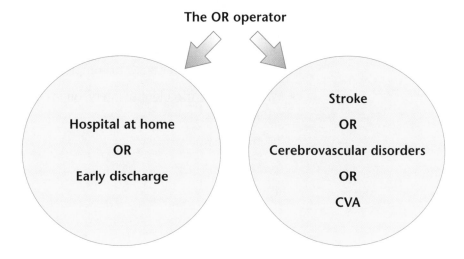

By combining two or more sets using OR, a new set will be created which contains all the documents in all the selected sets (with duplicates eliminated). This is also known as the *union* of the sets. In this example, using the OR operator will retrieve any article which mentions hospital at home or early discharge.

The AND operator

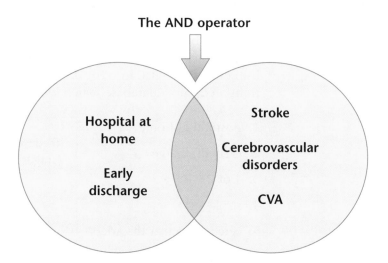

By combining two or more sets using AND, a new (shaded) set will be created which contains only those documents that the selected sets had in common (with duplicates eliminated). This is also known as the *intersection* of the sets. In this case AND will retrieve the subset of articles which mention hospital at home or early discharge and also mention stroke, cerebrovascular disorder or CVA.

Task 5.4 BOOLEAN OPERATORS

Draw a Venn diagram to represent how you would combine the terms for the following question. Use the synonyms and MESH headings you identified in Tasks 5.1 and 5.2 to complete the diagram.

→ What <u>non-pharmacological interventions</u> are effective in treating <u>arthritis</u>?

Stage 6: Reviewing results and refining your search

You may be wondering how the Venn diagram fits into a database search. Each term (both subject heading and synonyms if you are using them) is typed into the database separately. The Venn diagram is translated into a database search, which will look something like this:

1. hospital at home

2. early discharge

3. 1 or 2

     To describe the intervention (stages 1–3)

4. stroke

5. cerebrovascular disorders

6. 4 or 5

     To describe the condition (stages 4–6)

7. 3 and 6   To combine the two concepts

At each stage you can check the results to find out if particular terms are retrieving the desired results. You can also check the final result. If a term is causing a problem or you have retrieved too many studies you can easily refine the search.

For example, if you found that early discharge was giving you too many irrelevant results you could change the search by adding the line:

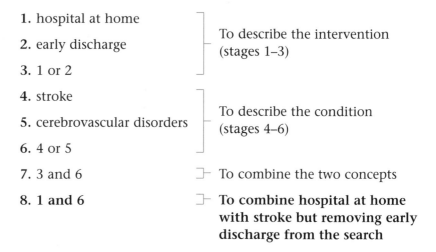

1. hospital at home

2. early discharge

3. 1 or 2

    To describe the intervention (stages 1–3)

4. stroke

5. cerebrovascular disorders

6. 4 or 5

    To describe the condition (stages 4–6)

7. 3 and 6   To combine the two concepts

8. 1 and 6   **To combine hospital at home with stroke but removing early discharge from the search**

This would combine the term hospital at home with the combined terms for stroke, but would exclude the term early discharge.

If this gave you too many articles you could then use the limit features to reduce them further. For example, you could limit to systematic reviews or randomised controlled trials. If the database software does not have limit features you could add a term to describe systematic reviews.

1. hospital at home

2. early discharge

3. 1 or 2

4. stroke

5. cerebrovascular disorders

6. 4 or 5

7. 3 and 6

8. 1 and 6

9. systematic review*   Retrieves systematic review, reviews or reviewing

10. 8 and 9   **To limit the original search to systematic reviews**

This would retrieve systematic reviews relating to hospital at home schemes for stroke.

KEY POINTS

❑ A search should be broken down into stages including clarifying the question and identifying terms for searching.

❑ A systematic approach will make the search process much easier and more effective. Searching on index terms is usually the most effective way of retrieving relevant articles, but you may need to search free text to ensure your search is comprehensive.

❑ Search terms should be combined using Boolean operators.

❑ Building the search in stages allows you to change your search in view of the results.

The process of carrying out a search should become much clearer once you have completed the practical exercises. You may wish to reread the relevant chapters as you are working through the practical exercises or revisit the whole section on completion of the practical exercises.

? QUIZ

1. What are the two ways of searching to ensure your results are comprehensive and/or overcome indexing problems?

   1.

   2.

2. Which Boolean operator allows you to obtain the intersection of two sets?

3. If you retrieve too many articles, what can you do?

SUGGESTED ANSWERS

Task 5.1: Suggested answers

List two MESH headings to describe each of the concepts in the question below.

→ What <u>non-pharmacological interventions</u> are effective in treating <u>arthritis</u>?

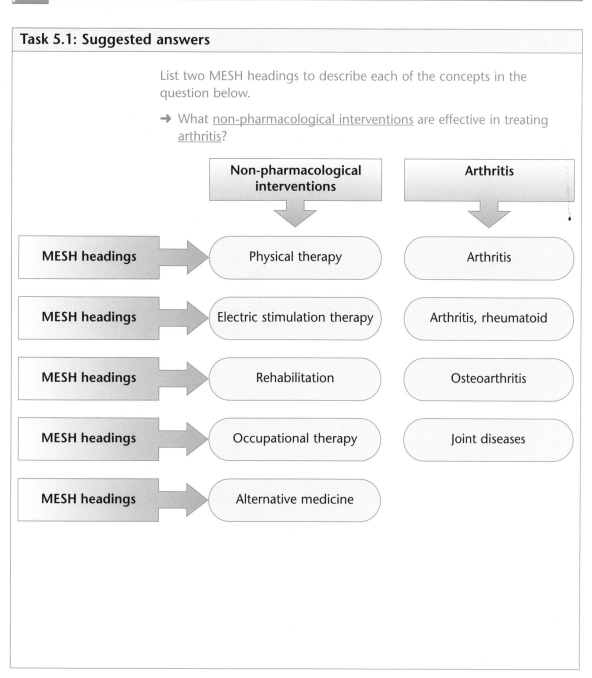

You may have found others; these are a selection of possibly relevant MESH headings.

Task 5.2: Suggested answers

Identify a range of synonyms to describe the concepts in the following question:

→ What <u>non-pharmacological interventions</u> are effective in treating <u>arthritis</u>?

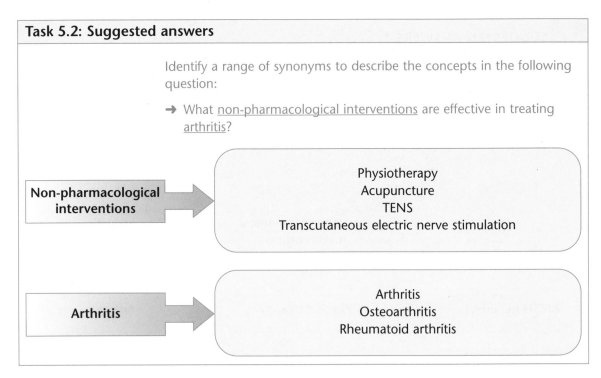

Non-pharmacological interventions	Physiotherapy Acupuncture TENS Transcutaneous electric nerve stimulation
Arthritis	Arthritis Osteoarthritis Rheumatoid arthritis

You may have thought of other synonyms.

Task 5.3: Suggested answers

Revisit the synonyms you identified in Task 5.2. Highlight any terms where you could use truncation or wildcard symbols and indicate where you would place the symbol. Remember if you put the truncation symbol too early, you may retrieve lots of irrelevant information.

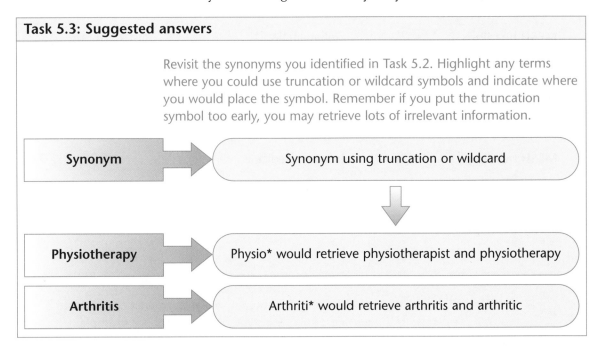

Synonym	Synonym using truncation or wildcard
Physiotherapy	Physio* would retrieve physiotherapist and physiotherapy
Arthritis	Arthriti* would retrieve arthritis and arthritic

For the examples above there were no relevant wildcards. There may have been in your suggestions.

Task 5.4: Suggested answers

Draw a Venn diagram to represent how you would combine the terms for the following question. Use the synonyms and MESH headings you identified in Tasks 5.1 and 5.2 to complete the diagram.

→ What <u>non-pharmacological interventions</u> are effective in treating <u>arthritis</u>?

Physical therapy OR alternative medicine OR TENS OR rehabilit* OR physiotherapy

Arthritis OR joint disease OR rheumatoid arthritis OR arthritis, rheumatoid

Quiz: Suggested answers

1. What are the two ways of searching to ensure your results are comprehensive and/or overcome indexing problems?

   1. Using MESH (keywords, subject headings).
   2. Searching free text.

2. Which Boolean operator allows you to obtain the intersection of two sets?

   AND allows you to retrieve articles with both (or all) your concepts, in effect reducing the number of articles.

3. If you retrieve too many articles, what can you do?

   Use the limit function, if available, to limit or restrict to a certain publication type or age group, for example. Alternatively add another concept on to restrict your search strategy.

CHAPTER 6

Conclusions and final tips

AIM

This chapter aims to draw together the lessons learned so far, and provide a few final tips on how to make searching the literature work for you.

CONCLUSION AND FINAL TIPS

Literature searching can be a complex business. However, by following the advice in this workbook, you will now have a structure and method of working which will enable you to search for information in a more efficient and effective way. Before highlighting a few key areas to bear in mind when searching, let's revisit the exercise at the beginning of this workbook to assess your attitudes and approaches to searching for information.

Concluding task ATTITUDES TO SEARCHING

In the Introduction to this workbook, a number of phrases were presented which may have encapsulated your approach to searching. The phrases are reproduced below. Write down your responses to the phrases now and compare these with your thoughts at the beginning of this workbook.

'I just sat down at the computer and did the search ...'

'I usually just search MEDLINE ...'

'I only use the Internet ...'

'I don't bother searching, I just ask a colleague ...'

'Every time I search I get loads of irrelevant references ...'

'I know my field and nothing has been published in this area ...'

MAKING YOUR SEARCH STRATEGY WORK FOR YOU

In the preceding chapters you were introduced to some of the tools, techniques and resources you may find helpful when undertaking a literature search. The techniques are transferable across electronic and printed resources, and should assist you in undertaking efficient and effective literature searches in the future. Here are a few final tips on getting the most out of your searches for information.

Be clear about what you are searching for

Consider the questions presented in Chapter 4. This will enable you to clarify the scope of the information you are searching for, and the opportunities and constraints in terms of the resources available to you.

Consider your sources

Consider the range of sources available to you, either locally in your library and information service, through professional organisations, or via the Internet. Then identify which sources are most likely to be appropriate in meeting your information need. Section 1 of this workbook should help clarify your thinking here. Once an appropriate resource has been identified, use the features of that resource to search it in the most effective way. For example, if searching an electronic database, consider using the thesaurus and synonyms to develop your search, and combine terms using Boolean operators. If searching the Internet, consider using quality assessed gateway and directory services as a first point of access. Always critically appraise the information you retrieve.

Be methodical

By using the techniques of developing your search question (Chapter 4), identifying the most appropriate resources you have access to (Chapters 1 and 2), and structuring your search strategy (Chapter 5), you can be confident about the thoroughness of your search process.

Be realistic

No matter how long you spend on developing and undertaking your search, no strategy is likely to be perfect. Searching is an iterative process. Be responsive to the types of information you retrieve, and be willing to adopt an alternative approach if you are not finding the materials you require. On the other hand, even if you do retrieve a large quantity of literature, whether from a single or multiple sources, this does not mean you have found everything published on a subject. Finally, bear in mind that in some cases a simple search of one resource is all that is necessary.

Expanding your search

When searching for information, you may find you need to expand your search; for example, if you are not retrieving relevant information. Consider alternative synonyms, perhaps by brainstorming your topic with friends or colleagues. If appropriate, search for known items and see how they are indexed, or recheck the thesaurus to identify additional search terms. If you have already identified useful materials, check any references cited as a way of identifying additional materials.

Limiting your search

If you retrieve too much information, consider refining your search question, perhaps by reducing the number of ideas or concepts covered. You might also use limits on your search, such as only searching within a particular time frame, or for materials published in a specific language. Some database packages have a limit function to enable you to do this more easily. Check the help function for details.

Save your thoughts

As you develop your search strategy, make a note of why you include some search terms, but not others. It may seem obvious to you now, but you can almost guarantee that by the time you revisit your search or write up your research your thought process will be less clear.

Save your search strategy

When you reach the end of a particular searching session, save a copy of your search strategy. Then, if you come to rerun the search, or wish to refine it based on your analysis of the papers retrieved, you will not have to retype it. You are also unlikely to remember all the terms you used previously. Some database packages have a function to allow you to do this easily and then rerun the search at a later date. For others, and for Internet searching, you will need to keep a written record of your search strategy.

Use help whenever necessary

Help exists in various forms such as the database help screen, colleagues, a librarian or simply by rereading this workbook. Remember that different databases and organisations use different software, so it is advisable to check the help menu to familiarise yourself with commands before you start your search. Alternatively, two heads can often be better than one in identifying search terms, so speak to colleagues about their experiences of using a particular database, or ask your local librarian. By combining your subject knowledge with their searching skills you can have a very strong team! Be aware of, and use, any sources of help that might be available.

KEY POINTS	
	❏ Literature searching is a skill that can be developed over time.
	❏ At first glance the depth of information presented in this workbook may seem daunting, but by approaching this book, much as you will your search, in a systematic and rigorous way, your skill and confidence will increase with each step. Good luck!

SUGGESTED ANSWERS

Concluding task: Suggested answers

The phrases presented at the beginning of this workbook, and at the beginning of this chapter, will shape your literature searches. The sample answers presented here provide an insight into how these statements might shape the type of information you retrieve.

'I just sat down at the computer and did the search ...'

> When searching for research evidence, it is important to tightly define the information you are looking for, and search a range of sources to ensure that you have obtained a good overview of the information available. Considering these issues before approaching the search will make your search more effective and you are less likely to get side-tracked or overwhelmed as you go along. Further details on these areas can be found in Section 1 on sources of information, and in Chapters 4 and 5 on search techniques, including defining your search question.

'I usually just search MEDLINE ...'

> Depending on your reason for searching, it may be appropriate to restrict your literature search to a single source: for example, if you are simply searching to obtain a couple of background papers for a presentation, or to support a point in a journal paper you are writing. However, if you are conducting a more in-depth literature review, you will probably need to search a range of information sources. This might mean using journal papers and reports from professional associations. Alternatively, you may include multiple database searches covering a variety of different topic areas, e.g. a biomedical database, a sociological database and a psychological database. The important thing to remember is to tailor your range of sources to best meet your information need. Further details can be found in Section 1 on sources of information.

'I only use the Internet ...'

Depending on your reason for searching, it may be appropriate to restrict your literature search to a single source. The Internet can provide access to many sources and to information on all kinds of topics, of varying quality and usefulness. Technological developments have made it possible for anyone to put information on the Internet. It can be difficult to know whether a site is authoritative or not. By using some of the tools and techniques listed in Chapter 3, ''The Internet ', and by critically appraising the information you access (in much the same way as you would other types of information), you can have increased confidence in the quality of the information.

'I don't bother searching, I just ask a colleague ...'

Colleagues can be helpful in providing you with an answer to a question quickly. However, as with all sources of information, it is important to evaluate the quality and evidence base of the information provided. That said, colleagues can be valuable in signposting alternative sources of information.

'Every time I search I get loads of irrelevant references ...'

If you retrieve too much information, you may need to consider refining your search question, perhaps by reducing the number of concepts covered, or by limiting your search to a particular time frame or language. Searching using MESH headings or keywords will ensure that the more relevant articles are retrieved. Further details about these techniques are included in Chapters 4 and 5 on search techniques.

'I know my field and nothing has been published in this area ...'

Although you may be familiar with the literature in your area, you may be surprised by the amount of additional information available even in a highly specialised area. By using the search techniques described in Chapters 4 and 5 and the resources highlighted in Chapters 1, 2 and 3, you can work with increased confidence knowing that you have a good overview of the information available in your subject area.

PRACTICAL EXERCISES

7. Practical exercises   81
8. MEDLINE: Ovid interface   83
9. MEDLINE: SilverPlatter interface   96
10. CINAHL: Ovid interface   109
11. CINAHL: SilverPlatter interface   122
12. Searching the Internet for healthcare information   135
13. Searching the National Electronic Library for Health (NeLH)   147

Practical exercises

This section aims to give you the opportunity to practise the techniques described earlier in the workbook using some of the sources outlined in Section 1.

There are many databases available to search and it would have been impossible to design practical exercises for all databases. The techniques described in the workbook are transferable across all sources; for illustration purposes the practical section focuses on MEDLINE, CINAHL, the Internet and the National Electronic Library for Health (NeLH), as these are widely available and relevant for a large number of health service professionals. Users of the workbook are encouraged to repeat the exercises using sources available to them in order to increase their skills and to understand the different material covered by different sources of information.

MEDLINE and CINAHL are available via a number of interfaces. Two of the most common are Ovid and SilverPlatter; exercises for both interfaces have been included here. Details of a PubMed tutorial are included below.

Before beginning the practical section, it is necessary to find out how you access these databases and the Internet in your organisation, and the software interface used. You may also need to obtain passwords. Your library or IT department should be able to help here.

Please note resources located on the Internet are constantly changing and electronic databases are frequently updated. The answers given in this section therefore were correct at the time of writing.

Other practical guides/tutorials

PubMed

PubMed is a free MEDLINE service; it is available via the Internet and the NeLH. An interactive tutorial is available from the PubMed home page:

www.ncbi.nlm.nih.gov/entrez/query.fcgi

Clinical databases provided on the National Electronic Library for Health

Clinical databases that can be accessed via NeLH are listed in Table 1 (pages 9–10). Guides to using them are available at:

http://nhs.dialog.com/Forms/Help%20Pages.htm#

Internet Detective

An interactive tutorial on evaluating the quality of Internet resources:

www.sosig.ac.uk/desire/internet-detective.html

Tonic

Online interactive web course introducing beginners to the Internet. Step-by-step practical guidance on major Internet topics:

www.netskills.ac.uk/TonicNG/cgi/sesame?tng

Virtual Training Suite

A set of teach-yourself subject based tutorials on searching the Internet:

www.vts.rdn.ac.uk

CHAPTER 8

MEDLINE: Ovid interface

Before beginning these practical exercises, ensure that you know how to log on to MEDLINE and that you have the appropriate passwords.

Once you have done this, log on to MEDLINE. Select 'MEDLINE 1966 to present'.

The exercises below introduce you to the concepts of literature searching, and guide you through developing a search. Although this example may not be of interest to you, it is useful to work through the exercises to learn the techniques. An opportunity to practise a search on a topic of interest to you is given at the end of the exercises.

Suggested answers, where appropriate, can be found on pages 90–95.

SEARCHING FOR A KNOWN ITEM

1. Find an article by Jenny Popay about qualitative research, write down the whole reference. Look at the complete record to see how it is laid out and the MESH/subject headings that have been used to describe the article.

Reference

MESH headings

SEARCHING FOR A SUBJECT

The following exercises will show you how to develop a search on the effectiveness of pressure-relieving mattresses on pressure sores.

Using MESH/subject headings

Searching using MESH/subject headings is a means of ensuring you obtain the information most relevant to your topic of interest.

1. What is the MESH/subject heading for pressure sores? Carry out a search on this heading.

2. What is the term higher up the tree (the broader term) for pressure sores?

3. What are the other term(s) at the same point in the hierarchy as the term for pressure sores?

4. Carry out a search for all types of skin ulcers. What function allows you to do this easily?

5. Compare the results of the search for all types of skin ulcers against that for decubitus ulcers. What changes when you broaden the search? (Note: This may vary from topic to topic.) What are the implications of this?

6. What is the MESH/subject heading for mattresses?

Combining terms

In order to find articles relating to mattresses and pressure sores it is necessary to combine these two concepts.

1. Combine the term 'decubitus ulcer' with 'beds'. Ensure you use the 'AND' Boolean operator to obtain the intersection of the two concepts.

2. Check the results. You should have retrieved articles discussing pressure sores and mattresses. However, you will probably have too many to look through and they are not restricted to those discussing the effectiveness.

3. Use the limit function to restrict the results to the following publication types: 'meta analysis', 'randomised controlled trial', 'review, academic', 'review literature'.

This will restrict the results to randomised controlled trials and reviews (hopefully summarising or testing the effectiveness of the mattresses in relation to pressure sores).

4. Note the other limit features that could have been used.

5. Check the results. Print out or save one or two of the most relevant articles.

6. Save the search strategy.

Searching free text

Although searching on MESH/subject headings is effective in identifying the majority of relevant literature on a database, it is also possible to miss relevant articles. Before expanding the search, practise using the 'truncation' and 'wildcard' techniques. *To search 'free text' remember to ensure that the 'map to subject heading' box is NOT ticked.*

Truncation

1. Type the following terms into MEDLINE to see how the truncation function works.

> Asthma$
> Respir$
> Osteo$

Display the articles retrieved. The phrase that you entered will be highlighted in bold. Check to see if articles on subjects you expected were retrieved.

Wildcards

The wildcard character (?) replaces 1 or 0 characters and can be used to retrieve alternative spellings. This is particularly useful to obtain articles with either English or American spellings.

1. Try using the wildcard character for the following words:

> Aging/Ageing
> Organisation/Organization
> Pediatric/Paediatric

2. Note the number of articles retrieved for each variation of the spelling. Think of the effect that this would have on the information retrieved if you only searched for one variation of the spelling.

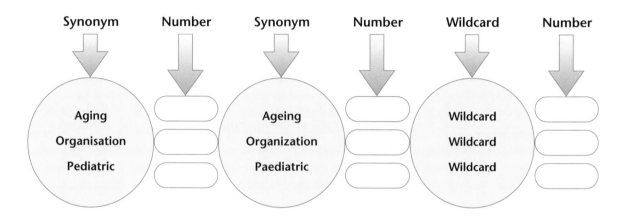

Synonym	Number	Synonym	Number	Wildcard	Number
Aging		Ageing		Wildcard	
Organisation		Organization		Wildcard	
Pediatric		Paediatric		Wildcard	

In Ovid MEDLINE there must be more than one letter in front of the wildcard character. Therefore you will have had problems with paediatric. To overcome this problem you need to search on both variations of the spelling.

To continue our pressure sore example:

3. Type in the following words that can also be used to describe pressure sores and mattresses.

> Pressure sore$
> Wound$
> Mattress$

Add these terms to your search strategy by:

4. Combining the terms relating to pressure sores, using the 'OR' Boolean operator.

5. Combining the terms relating to mattresses and beds using the 'OR' Boolean operator.

6. Combining the two concepts together using the 'AND' Boolean operator.

Your search will probably look something like this:

1. decubitus ulcer
2. beds
3. 1 AND 2
4. pressure sore$
5. wound$
6. mattress$
7. 1 OR 4 OR 5
8. 2 OR 6
9. 7 AND 8

7. Compare the results of this search with those of your earlier search (see 'Combining terms' above, point 2). What is the difference?

8. Limit this search to randomised controlled trials and systematic reviews.

9. Compare results with those of the earlier limited search (see 'Combining terms' above, point 3).

10. Check the results and print out one or two of the most relevant references.

11. Save your search strategy.

This is a basic introduction to building up a search strategy. Sometimes the effects of adding synonyms or using limit features are more dramatic than at other times. Try the same approach with different topic areas to see what happens.

SEARCHING FOR A TOPIC OF INTEREST TO YOU

Think of a topic of interest to you and carry out a literature search on MEDLINE for information relating to that topic.

The relevant steps are outlined to get you started.

Step One:
Phrase this idea in a manageable question.

Step Two:
Identify the important components.

Step Three:
Look up relevant MESH/subject headings – and perform a search on these MESH/subject headings.

Step Four:
Think of alternative synonyms to describe these concepts – and carry out searches on them (remember to use truncation and wildcards where appropriate).

Step Five:
Combine the concepts using Boolean operators.

Step Six:
Apply limits or refine the search as necessary.

REPEATING THE SEARCH ON ANOTHER DATABASE

Restricting a search to one database could miss a significant body of evidence.

Repeat either the 'pressure sores' search or the one on a topic of your own choosing using a different database available to you. Try and use the most appropriate database for your topic area.

Compare the results you obtained from this database with those obtained from CINAHL. Was there a large overlap? Were the same key papers retrieved?

Note: If the database you choose uses different software you may have to use different truncation and wildcard symbols. Check the help screens before starting your search.

SUGGESTED ANSWERS

SEARCHING FOR A KNOWN ITEM

1. Find an article by Jenny Popay about qualitative research, write down the whole reference. Look at the complete record to see how it is laid out and the MESH/subject headings that have been used to describe the article.

Reference ⟶ Popay J. Rogers A. Williams G. Rationale and standards for the systematic review of qualitative research in health services research. *Qualitative Health Research 8(3): 341–351, 1998.*

MESH headings ⟶ MESH/subject headings:
'evaluation studies', 'health services research', 'human', 'quality of health care', 'research design'

How to find the answer
Click on the author button. Type 'Popay, J' in the search box, click on 'perform search'. Scroll down the possibilities and click in the box next to the correct name. Click on 'perform search'. You can either scroll down the results (if there are a small number) or return to the main search screen and search for the word 'qualitative'. Click on the 'combine' button and click in the boxes next to the lines you wish to combine. Check that 'combine selections with' is set to the 'AND' Boolean operator, and click on 'continue'. Click on 'display' to see the records that have been retrieved.

Click on 'complete record' to see the full bibliographic records, including the MESH/subject headings.

SEARCHING FOR A SUBJECT

Developing a search on the effectiveness of pressure-relieving mattresses on pressure sores.

Using MESH/subject headings

1. What is the MESH/subject heading for pressure sores?

> Decubitus ulcer

How to find the answer
Type the phrase 'pressure sores' into the search box. Ensure that 'map to subject heading' is ticked. This will give you a list of potentially relevant subject headings. Select the one you think is most appropriate. Click on the 'I' (information icon) to read the definition to confirm it relates to pressure sores.

2. What is the term higher up in the hierarchy (the broader term for pressure sores)?

> Skin ulcer

How to find the answer
Click on the term 'decubitus ulcer'. This displays the term and its place in the hierarchy of terms. (You may need to scroll down the screen to find the term.) The term higher in the hierarchy of decubitus ulcer (above and to the left) is 'skin ulcer'.

Answers continue

3. What are the term(s) at the same point in the hierarchy as the term for pressure sores?

> Leg ulcer and pyoderma gangrenosum

How to find the answer
In the hierarchy of 'skin ulcer', there is a lower level of indexing (displayed below and to the right of 'skin ulcer'). This includes 'decubitus ulcer'. There are two other terms on the same level – 'leg ulcer' and 'pyoderma gangrenosum'.

4. Carry out a search for all types of skin ulcers. What function allows you to do this easily?

> Explode

How to find the answer
Click on the box next to 'skin ulcer'. There are two columns of boxes to the right of the screen. The first of these boxes is the 'explode' box (if you scroll to the top of the screen, the columns are labelled 'explode' and 'focus'). Click in the 'explode' box. This will search for all types of skin ulcer: the broader term of 'skin ulcer' and the lower levels of indexing. In this case, this includes 'decubitus ulcer', 'leg ulcer' and 'pyoderma gangrenosum'.

5. Compare the results of the search for all type of skin ulcers against that for decubitus ulcers. What happens when you broaden the search? (Note: This may vary from topic to topic.) What are the implications of this?

> A larger number of records are retrieved when the explode function is used. This can be useful if you wish to search a subject comprehensively. However, in this instance, only literature related to pressure sores is wanted. An 'exploded' search in not therefore necessary, as many of the records are likely to be irrelevant because the search includes other types of ulcers.

6. What is the MESH heading for mattresses?

Beds

How to find the answer
Type the phrase 'mattresses' into the search box. Ensure that 'map to subject heading' is ticked. This will give you a list of potentially relevant subject headings. Select the one you think is most appropriate. Click on the 'I' (information icon) to read the definition to confirm it relates to mattresses.

Combining terms

1. Combine the terms 'decubitus ulcer' and 'beds'. Ensure you use the 'AND' Boolean operator to obtain the intersection of the two terms.

How to find the answer
Click on the 'combine' button and click in the boxes next to the lines you wish to combine – 'decubitus ulcer' and 'beds'. Check that 'combine selections with' is set to the 'AND' Boolean operator, and click on 'continue'. This will search for papers that mention the terms 'decubitus ulcer' and 'beds'.

Click on 'display' to see the records that have been retrieved.

3. Use the limit function to restrict the results to the following publication types: 'meta-analysis', 'randomised controlled trial', 'review, academic' and 'review literature'.

How to find the answer
Click on the 'limit' button. Scroll down the screen until you see a box entitled 'Publication Types'. Use the scroll button of this box to find the limit fields you want, e.g. 'meta analysis', 'randomised controlled trial', 'review, academic' and 'review literature'. Hold down the 'Ctrl' key and click the button on the mouse to select more than one limit field at a time. Click on the 'limit search' button in the top left hand corner of the screen. The limit will automatically be applied to the last search undertaken, unless you select an alternative search line.

4. Note the other limit features that could have been used.

> Age, animal types, language, publication year

How to find the answer
Click on the 'limit' button. There are a few limit features at the bottom of the screen. If you scroll further down the page you will see more limit options. Select the ones you want. Hold down the 'Ctrl' key and click the button on the mouse to select more than one limit field at a time.

Searching free text

Truncation

1. Type the following terms into MEDLINE to see how the truncation function works.

> Asthma$
> Respir$
> Osteo$

Display the articles retrieved. The phrase that you entered will be highlighted in bold. Check to see if articles on subjects you expected were retrieved.

> You should have retrieved articles with a variety of terms including: asthmatics, respiratory, respiration, osteoporosis, osteoarthritis etc.
>
> Note: If you truncate too early you will get irrelevant information. For example, if you were interested in osteoporosis it would be more useful to enter osteop$ rather than osteo$.

Wildcards

2. Note the number of articles retrieved for each variation of the spelling. Think of the effect that this would have on the information retrieved if you only searched for one variation of the spelling.

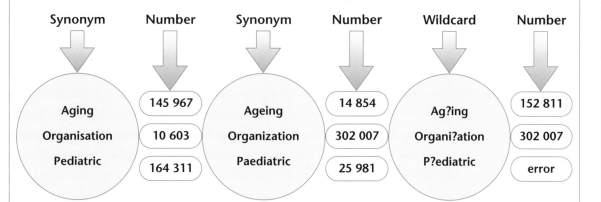

Synonym	Number	Synonym	Number	Wildcard	Number
Aging	145 967	Ageing	14 854	Ag?ing	152 811
Organisation	10 603	Organization	302 007	Organi?ation	302 007
Pediatric	164 311	Paediatric	25 981	P?ediatric	error

In Ovid MEDLINE there must be more than one letter in front of the wildcard character. If this is not the case, an error message is returned indicating an improper placement of the wildcard character and inviting you to try again. Therefore you will have had problems with paediatric. To overcome this problem you need to search on both variations of the spelling.

1. pediatric
2. paediatric
3. 1 OR 2

7. Compare the results of this search with those of your earlier search. What is the difference?

A larger number of records are retrieved when the explode function is used. This can be useful if you wish to search a subject comprehensively. However, in this instance, only literature related to pressure sores is wanted. An 'exploded' search is not therefore necessary, as many of the records are likely to be irrelevant because the search includes other types of ulcers.

MEDLINE: SilverPlatter interface (WebSPIRS or WinSPIRS)

Before beginning these practical exercises, ensure that you know how to log on to MEDLINE in your organisation and that you have the appropriate passwords.

Once you have done this, log on to MEDLINE.

The exercises below introduce you to the concepts of literature searching, and guide you through developing a search. Although this example may not be of interest to you, it is useful to work through the exercises to learn the techniques. An opportunity to practise a search on a topic of interest to you is given at the end of the exercises.

Suggested answers, where appropriate, can be found on pages 103–108.

SEARCHING FOR A KNOWN ITEM

1. Find an article by Jenny Popay about qualitative research written in 1998. Write down the whole reference. Look at the complete record to see how it is laid out and the subject/thesaurus terms (MJME and MNME – major MESH and minor MESH terms) that have been used to describe the article.

Reference ➤

Thesaurus terms ➤

SEARCHING FOR A SUBJECT

The following exercises will show you how to develop a search on the effectiveness of pressure-relieving mattresses on pressure sores.

Using subject/thesaurus terms

Searching using subject/thesaurus terms is a means of ensuring you obtain the information most relevant to your topic of interest.

1. What is the subject/thesaurus term for pressure sores? Carry out a search on this subject/thesaurus term.

2. What is the term higher up the hierarchy (the broader term) for pressure sores?

3. What are the other term(s) at the same point in the hierarchy as the term for pressure sores?

4. Carry out a search for all types of skin ulcers. What function allows you to do this easily?

5. Compare the results of the search for all types of skin ulcers against that for decubitus ulcers. What happens when you broaden the search? (Note: This may vary from topic to topic.) What are the implications of this?

6. What is the subject/thesaurus term for mattresses?

Combining terms

In order to find articles relating to mattresses and pressure sores it is necessary to combine these two concepts.

1. Combine the term 'decubitus-ulcer' with 'beds'. Ensure you use the 'AND' Boolean operator to obtain the intersection of the two concepts.

2. Check the results. You should have retrieved articles discussing pressure sores and mattresses. However, you will probably have too many to look through and they are not restricted to those discussing effectiveness.

3. Use the limit function to restrict the results to the following publication types: 'meta-analysis', 'randomised-controlled-trial', 'review-academic', 'review-literature'.

This will restrict the results to randomised controlled trials and reviews (hopefully summarising or testing the effectiveness of the mattresses in relation to pressure sores).

4. Note the other limit features that could have been used.

5. Check the results. Print out or save one or two of the most relevant articles.

6. Save the search strategy.

Searching free text

Although searching on subject/thesaurus terms is effective in identifying the majority of relevant literature on a database, it is also possible to miss relevant articles. Before expanding the search, practise using the 'truncation' and 'wildcard' techniques.

Truncation

1. Type the following terms into MEDLINE to see how the truncation function works.

> Asthma*
> Respir*
> Osteo*

Display the articles retrieved. The phrase that you entered will be highlighted in bold. Check to see if articles on subjects you expected were retrieved.

Wildcards

The wildcard character (?) replaces 1 or 0 characters and can be used to retrieve alternative spellings. This is particularly useful to obtain articles with either English or American spellings.

1. Try using the wildcard character for the following words:

> Aging/Ageing
> Organisation/Organization
> Pediatric/Paediatric

2. Note the number of articles retrieved for each variation of the spelling. Think of the effect that this would have on the information retrieved if you only searched for one variation of the spelling.

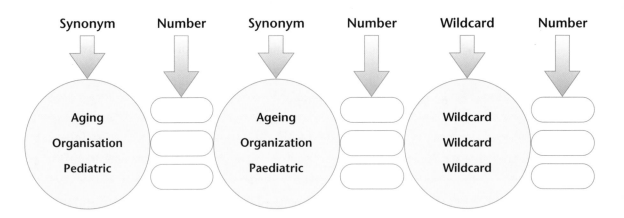

To continue our pressure sore example:

3. Type in the following words that can also be used to describe pressure sores and mattresses.

> Pressure sore*
> Wound*
> Mattress*

Add these terms to your search strategy by:

4. Combining the terms relating to pressure sores, using the 'OR' Boolean operator.

5. Combining the terms relating to mattresses and beds, using the 'OR' Boolean operator.

6. Combining the two concepts together, using the 'AND' Boolean operator.

Your search will probably look something like this:

9. 7 AND 8
8. 2 OR 6
7. 1 OR 4 OR 5
6. mattress*
5. wound*
4. pressure sore*
3. 1 AND 2
2. beds
1. decubitus-ulcer

7. Compare the results of this search with those of your earlier search (see 'Combining terms' above, point 2). What is the difference?

8. Limit this search to randomized controlled trials and systematic reviews.

9. Compare results with those of the earlier limited search (see 'Combining terms' above, point 3).

10. Check the results and print out one or two of the most relevant references.

11. Save your search strategy.

This is a basic introduction to building up a search strategy. Sometimes the effects of adding synonyms or using limit features are more dramatic than at other times. Try the same approach with different topic areas to see what happens.

SEARCHING FOR A TOPIC OF INTEREST TO YOU

Think of a topic of interest to you and carry out a literature search on MEDLINE for information relating to that topic.

The relevant steps are outlined to get you started.

Step One:
Phrase this idea in a manageable question.

Step Two:
Identify the important components.

Step Three:
Look up relevant subject/thesaurus terms – and perform a search on these subject/thesaurus terms.

Step Four
Think of alternative synonyms to describe these concepts – and carry out searches on them (remember to use truncation and wildcards where appropriate).

Step Five:
Combine the concepts using Boolean operators.

Step Six:
Apply limits or refine the search as necessary.

REPEATING THE SEARCH ON ANOTHER DATABASE

Restricting a search to one database could miss a significant body of evidence.

Repeat either the 'pressure sores' search or the one on a topic of your own choosing using a different database available to you. Try and use the most appropriate database for your topic area.

Compare the results you obtained from this database with those obtained from CINAHL. Was there a large overlap? Were the same key papers retrieved?

Note: If the database you choose uses different software you may have to use different truncation and wildcard symbols. Check the help screens before starting your searching.

SUGGESTED ANSWERS

SEARCHING FOR A KNOWN ITEM

1. Find an article by Jenny Popay about qualitative research. Write down the whole reference. Look at the complete record to see how it is laid out and the subject/thesaurus terms that have been used to describe the article.

Reference

> Popay J. Rogers A. Williams G. Rationale and standards for the systematic review of qualitative research in health services research. *Qualitative Health Research 8(3): 341–351, 1998.*

Thesaurus terms

> Subject/thesaurus terms:
> 'evaluation studies', 'health services research', 'quality of health care', 'research design'

How to find the answer
Click the author button. Type 'Popay J' in the search box, click on 'start search'. You can either scroll down the results (if there are a small number) or return to the main search screen and check the 'words anywhere' button and search for the word 'qualitative'. Return to the main search screen and click in the boxes next to the lines you wish to combine. Using the 'AND' Boolean operator, click on the 'combined checked' button to the left of the screen. This will search for papers which mention the word qualitative and the author J Popay.

Click on the record number to link to the complete record – this will allow you to see all fields in the record, including the subject/thesaurus terms (MJME/MNME).

Answers continue

SEARCHING FOR A SUBJECT

Developing a search on the effectiveness of pressure-relieving mattresses on pressure sores.

Using subject/thesaurus terms

1. What is the subject/thesaurus term for pressure sores?

> Decubitus-ulcer

How to find the answer
Click on the 'thesaurus' button on the right hand side of the screen. Type the phrase 'pressure sores' into the subject box. Click on 'go to subject'. This will give you a list of potentially relevant subject terms. Select the one you think is most appropriate. Click on the term and read the definition to confirm it relates to pressure sores.

2. What is the term higher up in the hierarchy (the broader term) for pressure sores?

> Skin-ulcer

How to find the answer
Broader and narrow terms are displayed on the same page as the definition for subject/thesaurus terms.

3. What are the other term(s) at the same point in the hierarchy as the term for pressure sores?

Leg-ulcer and pyoderma-gangrenosum

How to find the answer
Click on the broader term 'skin-ulcer'. This gives you more information about the term and its place in the hierarchy of terms. Narrower and broader terms are also listed. The term 'pressure-ulcer' is a narrower term of 'skin-ulcer', and appears on the same level as 'leg-ulcer' and 'pyoderma-gangrenosum'.

4. Carry out a search for all types of skin ulcers. What function allows you to do this easily?

Explode

How to find the answer
Click on 'skin-ulcer'. Look at the box at the top of the screen. Click on the 'explode subject' button, and then click on the 'explode checked subjects' button. This will search on terms in the subject/thesaurus term hierarchy that you have displayed. In this case all types of skin ulcer.

5. Compare the results of the search for all type of skin ulcers against that for decubitus ulcer. What happens when you broaden the search? (Note: This may vary from topic to topic.) What are the implications of this?

A larger number of records are retrieved when the explode function is used. This can be useful if you wish to search a subject comprehensively. However, in this instance, only literature related to pressure sores is wanted. An 'exploded' search in not therefore necessary, as many of the records are likely to be irrelevant because the search includes other types of ulcers.

6. What is the subject/thesaurus term for mattresses?

> Beds

How to find the answer
Click on the 'thesaurus' button on the right hand side of the screen. Type the phrase 'mattresses' into the subject box. Click on 'go to subject'. This will give you a list of potentially relevant subject/thesaurus terms. Select the one you think is most appropriate. Click on the term and read the definition to confirm it relates to mattresses.

Combining terms

1. Combine the terms 'decubitus-ulcer' and 'beds'. Ensure you use the 'AND' Boolean operator to obtain the intersection of the two terms.

How to find the answer
Return to the main search screen and click in the boxes next to the lines you wish to combine – 'decubitus-ulcer' and 'beds'. Ensure the 'AND' Boolean operator is selected. Click on the 'combined checked' button to the left of the screen. This will search for papers that mention the word terms 'decubitus-ulcer' and 'beds'.

Click on 'display' to see the records that have been retrieved.

3. Use the limit function to restrict the results to the following publication types: 'meta-analysis', 'randomised-controlled-trial', 'review-academic' and 'review-literature'.

How to find the answer
Return to the main search screen and, on the left hand side of the screen, click in the button 'limit your search'. Scroll down the screen until you see a box entitled 'PT-Publication Type'. Use the scroll button of this box to find the limit fields you want, e.g. 'meta-analysis', 'randomised-controlled-trial', 'review-academic' and 'review-literature'. Hold down the 'Ctrl' key and click the button on the mouse. This will enable you to select more than one limit field at a time. Click on the 'set limits' button in the top right hand corner of the screen.

Now click in the box next to the search line you would like to apply the limit to, and click on the 're-type checked' button on the left of the screen. Click on the 'start search' button next to the search box.

4. Note the other limit features that could have been used.

> Age, country of publication, language, publication year

Searching free text

Truncation

1. Type the following terms into MEDLINE to see how the truncation function works.

> Asthma*
> Respir*
> Osteo*

Display the articles retrieved. The phrase that you entered will be highlighted in bold. Check to see if articles on subjects you expected were retrieved.

> You should have retrieved articles with a variety of terms including: asthmatics, respiratory, respiration, osteoporosis, osteoarthritis etc.
>
> Note: If you truncate too early you will get irrelevant information. For example, if you were interested in osteoporosis it would be more useful to enter osteop* rather than osteo*.

Wildcards

2. Note the number of articles retrieved for each variation of the spelling. Think of the effect that this would have on the information retrieved if you only searched for one variation of the spelling.

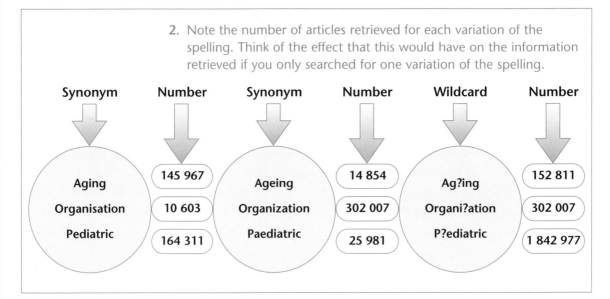

Synonym	Number	Synonym	Number	Wildcard	Number
Aging	145 967	Ageing	14 854	Ag?ing	152 811
Organisation	10 603	Organization	302 007	Organi?ation	302 007
Pediatric	164 311	Paediatric	25 981	P?ediatric	1 842 977

7. Compare the results of this search with those of your earlier search. What is the difference?

> You retrieve more articles and reduce the chance of missing potentially relevant records.

CHAPTER 10

CINAHL:
Ovid interface

Before beginning these practical exercises, ensure that you know how to log on to CINAHL and that you have the appropriate passwords.

Once you have done this, log on to CINAHL.

The exercises below introduce you to the concepts of literature searching, and guide you through developing a search. Although this example may not be of interest to you, it is useful to work through the exercises to learn the techniques. An opportunity to practise a search on a topic of interest to you is given at the end of the exercises.

Suggested answers, where appropriate, can be found on pages 116–121.

SEARCHING FOR A KNOWN ITEM

1. Find an article by Jenny Popay about qualitative research, write down the whole reference. Look at the complete record to see how it is laid out and the subject headings that have been used to describe the article.

Reference

Subject headings

SEARCHING FOR A SUBJECT

The following exercises will show you how to develop a search on the effectiveness of pressure-relieving mattresses on pressure sores.

Using subject headings

Searching using subject headings is a means of ensuring you obtain the information most relevant to your topic of interest.

1. What is the subject heading for pressure sores? Carry out a search on this heading.

2. What is the term higher up the tree (the broader term) for pressure sores?

3. What are the other term(s) at the same point in the hierarchy as the term for pressure sores?

4. Carry out a search for all types of skin ulcers. What function allows you to do this easily?

5. Compare the results of the search for all type of skin ulcers against that of pressure sores. What changes when you broaden the search? (Note: This may vary from topic to topic.) What are the implications of this?

6. What is the subject heading for mattresses?

Combining terms

In order to find articles relating to mattresses and pressure sores it is necessary to combine these two concepts.

1. Combine the term 'pressure ulcer' with 'beds and mattresses'. Ensure you use the 'AND' Boolean operator to obtain the intersection of the two concepts.

2. Check the results. You should have retrieved articles discussing pressure sores and mattresses. However, you will probably have too many to look through and they are not restricted to those discussing the effectiveness.

3. Use the limit function to restrict the results to the following publication types: 'clinical trial' and 'review'.

This will restrict the results to clinical trials and reviews (hopefully summarising or testing the effectiveness of the mattresses in relation to pressure sores).

4. Note the other limit features that could have been used.

5. Check the results. Print out or save one or two of the most relevant articles.

6. Save the search strategy.

Searching free text

Although searching on subject headings is effective in identifying the majority of relevant literature on a database, it is also possible to miss relevant articles. Before expanding the search, practise using the 'truncation' and 'wildcard' techniques. *To search 'free text' remember to ensure that the 'map to subject heading' box is NOT ticked.*

Truncation

1. Type the following terms into CINAHL to see how the truncation function works.

> Asthma$
> Respir$
> Osteo$

Display the articles retrieved. The phrase that you entered will be highlighted in bold. Check to see if articles on subjects you expected were retrieved.

Wildcards

The wildcard character (?) replaces 1 or 0 characters and can be used to retrieve alternative spellings. This is particularly useful to obtain articles with either English or American spellings.

1. Try using the wildcard character for the following words:

> Aging/Ageing
> Organisation/Organization
> Pediatric/Paediatric

2. Note the number of articles retrieved for each variation of the spelling. Think of the effect that this would have on the information retrieved if you only searched for one variation of the spelling.

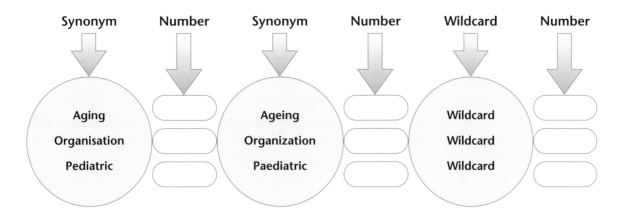

In Ovid CINAHL there must be more than one letter in front of the wildcard character. Therefore, you will have had problems with paediatric. To overcome this problem you need to search on both variations of the spelling.

To continue our pressure sore example:

3. Type in the following words that can also be used to describe pressure sores and mattresses.

    Pressure sore$
    Wound$
    Mattress$

Add these terms to your search strategy by:

4. Combining the terms relating to pressure sores, using the 'OR' Boolean operator.

5. Combining the terms relating to mattresses and beds using the 'OR' Boolean operator.

6. Combining the two concepts together using the 'AND' Boolean operator.

Your search will probably look something like this:

1. pressure ulcer
2. beds and mattresses
3. 1 AND 2
4. pressure sore$
5. wound$
6. mattress$
7. 1 OR 4 OR 5
8. 2 OR 6
9. 7 AND 8

7. Compare the results of this search with those of your earlier search (see 'Combining terms' above, point 2). What is the difference?

8. Limit this search to clinical trials, systematic reviews and reviews.

9. Compare results with those of the earlier limited search (see 'Combining terms' above, point 3).

10. Check the results and print out one or two of the most relevant references.

11. Save your search strategy.

This is a basic introduction to building up a search strategy. Sometimes the effects of adding synonyms or using limit features are more dramatic than at other times. Try the same approach with different topic areas to see what happens.

SEARCHING FOR A TOPIC OF INTEREST TO YOU

Think of a topic of interest to you and carry out a literature search on CINAHL for information relating to that topic.

The relevant steps are outlined to get you started.

Step One:
Phrase this idea in a manageable question.

Step Two:
Identify the important components.

Step Three:
Look up relevant subject headings – and perform a search on these headings.

Step Four:
Think of alternative synonyms to describe these concepts – and carry out searches on them (remember to use truncation and wildcards where appropriate).

Step Five:
Combine the concepts using Boolean operators.

Step Six:
Apply limits or refine search as necessary.

REPEATING THE SEARCH ON ANOTHER DATABASE

Restricting a search to one database could miss a significant body of evidence.

Repeat either of these searches on a different database available to you. Try and use the most appropriate database for your topic area.

Compare the results you obtained from this database with those obtained from MEDLINE. Was there a large overlap? Were the same key papers retrieved?

Note: If the database you choose uses different software you may have to use different truncation and wildcard symbols. Check the help screens before starting your search.

SUGGESTED ANSWERS

SEARCHING FOR A KNOWN ITEM

1. Find an article by Jenny Popay about qualitative research. Write down the whole reference. Look at the complete record to see how it is laid out and the subject headings that have been used to describe the article.

Reference

> Popay J. Rogers A. Williams G. Rationale and standards for the systematic review of qualitative research in health services research. *Qualitative Health Research 8(3): 341–351, 1998.*

Subject headings

> Subject headings:
> 'health services research', 'qualitative studies', 'systematic review'

How to find the answer
Click on the author button. Type 'Popay, J' in the search box, click on 'perform search'. Scroll down the possibilities and click in the box next to the correct name. Click on 'perform search'. You can either scroll down the results (if there are a small number) or return to the main search screen and search for the word 'qualitative'. Click on the 'combine' button and click in the boxes next to the lines you wish to combine. Check that 'combine selections with' is set to the 'AND' Boolean operator, and click on 'continue'. Click on 'display' to see the records that have been retrieved.

Click on 'complete record' to see the full bibliographic records, including the subject headings.

SEARCHING FOR A SUBJECT

Developing a search on the effectiveness of pressure-relieving mattresses on pressure sores.

Using subject headings

1. What is the subject heading for pressure sores?

> Pressure ulcer

How to find the answer
Type the phrase 'pressure sores' into the search box. Ensure that 'map to subject heading' is ticked. This will give you a list of potentially relevant subject headings. Select the one you think is most appropriate. Click on the 'I' (information icon) to read the definition to confirm it relates to pressure sores.

2. What is the term higher up in the hierarchy (the broader term for pressure sores)?

> Skin ulcer

How to find the answer
Click on the term 'pressure ulcer'. This displays the term and its place in the hierarchy of terms. (You may need to scroll down the screen to find the term.) The term higher in the hierarchy of pressure ulcer (above and to the left) is 'skin ulcer'.

Answers continue

3. What are the other term(s) at the same point in the hierarchy as the term for pressure sores?

> Leg ulcer and pyoderma gangrenosum

How to find the answer
In the hierarchy of 'skin ulcer', there is a lower level of indexing (displayed below and to the right of 'skin ulcer'). This includes 'pressure ulcer'. There are two other terms on the same level – 'leg ulcer' and 'pyoderma gangrenosum'.

4. Carry out a search for all types of skin ulcers. What function allows you to do this easily?

> Explode

How to find the answer
Click on the box next to 'skin ulcer'. There are two columns of boxes to the right of the screen. The first of these boxes is the 'explode' box (if you scroll to the top of the screen, the columns are labelled 'explode' and 'focus'). Click in the 'explode' box. This will search for all types of skin ulcer: the broader term of 'skin ulcer' and the lower levels of indexing. In this case, this includes 'pressure ulcer', 'leg ulcer' and 'pyoderma gangrenosum'.

5. Compare the results of the search for all type of skin ulcers against that for decubitus ulcer. What happens when you broaden the search? (Note: This may vary from topic to topic.) What are the implications of this?

> A larger number of records are retrieved when the explode function is used. This can be useful if you wish to search a subject comprehensively. However, in this instance, only literature related to pressure sores is wanted. An 'exploded' search in not therefore necessary, as many of the records are likely to be irrelevant because the search includes other types of ulcers.

6. What is the subject heading for mattresses?

> Beds and matresses

How to find the answer
Type the word 'mattresses' into the search box. Ensure that 'map to subject heading' is ticked. This will give you a list of potentially relevant subject headings. Select the one you think is most appropriate. Click on the 'I' (information icon) to read the definition to confirm it relates to mattresses.

Combining terms

1. Combine the terms 'pressure ulcer' and 'beds and mattresses'. Ensure you use the 'AND' Boolean operator to obtain the intersection of the two terms.

How to find the answer
Click on the 'combine' button and click in the boxes next to the lines you wish to combine – 'pressure ulcer' and 'beds and mattresses'. Check that 'combine selections with' is set to the 'AND' Boolean operator, and click on 'continue'. This will search for papers that mention the terms 'pressure ulcer' and 'beds and mattresses'.

Click on 'display' to see the records that have been retrieved.

3. Use the limit function to restrict the results to the following publication types: 'clinical trial' and 'review'.

How to find the answer
Click on the 'limit' button. Scroll down the screen until you see a box entitled 'Publication Types'. Use the scroll button of this box to find the limit fields you want, e.g. 'clinical trial' and 'review'. Hold down the 'Ctrl' key and click the button on the mouse to select more than one limit field at a time. Click on the 'limit search' button in the top left hand corner of the screen. The limit will automatically be applied to the last search undertaken, unless you select an alternative search line.

4. Note the other limit features that could have been used.

> Age, language, publication year

How to find the answer
Click on the 'limit' button. There are a few limit features at the bottom of the screen. If you scroll further down the page you will see more limit options. Select the ones you want. Hold down the 'Ctrl' key and click the button on the mouse to select more than one limit field at a time.

Searching free text

Truncation

1. Type the following terms into CINAHL to see how the truncation function works.

> Asthma$
> Respir$
> Osteo$

Display the articles retrieved. The phrase that you entered will be highlighted in bold. Check to see if articles on subjects you expected were retrieved.

> You should have retrieved articles with a variety of terms including: asthmatics, respiratory, respiration, osteoporosis, osteoarthritis etc.
>
> Note: If you truncate too early you will get irrelevant information. For example, if you were interested in osteoporosis it would be more useful to enter osteop$ rather than osteo$.

Wildcards

2. Note the number of articles retrieved for each variation of the spelling. Think of the effect that this would have on the information retrieved if you only searched for one variation of the spelling.

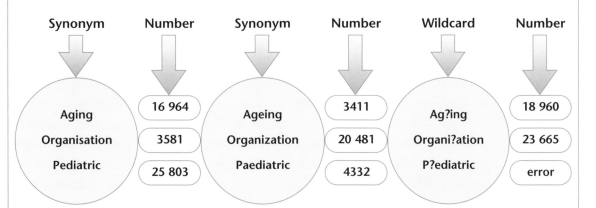

Synonym	Number	Synonym	Number	Wildcard	Number
Aging	16 964	Ageing	3411	Ag?ing	18 960
Organisation	3581	Organization	20 481	Organi?ation	23 665
Pediatric	25 803	Paediatric	4332	P?ediatric	error

In Ovid CINAHL there must be more than one letter in front of the wildcard character. If this is not the case, an error message is returned indicating an improper placement of the wildcard character and inviting you to try again. Therefore you will have had problems with paediatric. To overcome this problem you need to search on both variations of the spelling.

1. pediatric
2. paediatric
3. 1 OR 2

7. Compare the results of this search with those of your earlier search. What is the difference?

A larger number of records are retrieved when the explode function is used. This can be useful if you wish to search a subject comprehensively. However, in this instance, only literature related to pressure sores is wanted. An 'exploded' search is not therefore necessary, as many of the records are likely to be irrelevant because the search includes other types of ulcers.

CINAHL: SilverPlatter interface (WebSPIRS or WinSPIRS)

Before beginning these practical exercises, ensure that you know how to log on to CINAHL in your organisation and that you have the appropriate passwords.

Once you have done this, log on to CINAHL.

The exercises below introduce you to the concepts of literature searching, and guide you through developing a search. Although this example may not be of interest to you, it is useful to work through the exercises to learn the techniques. An opportunity to practise a search on a topic of interest to you is given at the end of the exercises.

Suggested answers, where appropriate, can be found on pages 129–134.

SEARCHING FOR A KNOWN ITEM

1. Find an article by Jenny Popay about qualitative research written in 1998. Write down the whole reference. Look at the complete record to see how it is laid out and the subject/thesaurus terms (MJ and MN – major and minor terms) that have been used to describe the article.

Reference

Thesaurus terms

SEARCHING FOR A SUBJECT

The following exercises will show you how to develop a search on the effectiveness of pressure-relieving mattresses on pressure sores.

Using subject/thesaurus terms

Searching using subject/thesaurus terms is a means of ensuring you obtain the information most relevant to your topic of interest.

1. What is the subject/thesaurus term for pressure sores? Carry out a search on this subject/thesaurus term.

2. What is the subject/thesaurus term higher up the hierarchy (the broader term) for pressure sores?

3. What are the other subject/thesaurus term(s) at the same point in the hierarchy as the subject/thesaurus term for pressure sores?

4. Carry out a search for all types of skin ulcers. What function allows you to do this easily?

5. Compare the results of the search for all types of skin ulcers against that for pressure ulcer. What happens when you broaden the search? (Note: This may vary from topic to topic.) What are the implications of this?

6. What is the subject/thesaurus term for mattresses?

Combining subject/thesaurus terms

In order to find articles relating to mattresses and pressure sores it is necessary to combine these two concepts.

1. Combine the subject/thesaurus term 'pressure-ulcer' with 'beds-and-mattresses'. Ensure you use the 'AND' Boolean operator to obtain the intersection of the two concepts.

2. Check the results. You should have retrieved articles discussing pressure sores and mattresses. However, you will probably have too many to look through and they are not restricted to those discussing effectiveness.

3. Use the limit function to restrict the results to the following document types: 'clinical-trial' and 'review'.

This will restrict the results to clinical trials and reviews (hopefully summarising or testing the effectiveness of the mattresses in relation to pressure sores).

4. Note the other limit features that could have been used.

5. Check the results. Print out or save one or two of the most relevant articles.

6. Save the search strategy.

Searching free text

Although searching on subject/thesaurus terms is effective in identifying the majority of relevant literature on a database, it is also possible to miss relevant articles. Before expanding the search, practise using the 'truncation' and 'wildcard' techniques.

Truncation

1. Type the following terms into CINAHL to see how the truncation function works.

    Asthma*
    Respir*
    Osteo*

Display the articles retrieved. The phrase that you entered will be highlighted in bold. Check to see if articles on subjects you expected were retrieved.

Wildcards

The wildcard character (?) replaces 1 or 0 characters and can be used to retrieve alternative spellings. This is particularly useful to obtain articles with either English or American spellings.

1. Try using the wildcard character for the following words:

    Aging/Ageing
    Organisation/Organization
    Pediatric/Paediatric

2. Note the number of articles retrieved for each variation of the spelling. Think of the effect that this would have on the information retrieved if you only searched for one variation of the spelling.

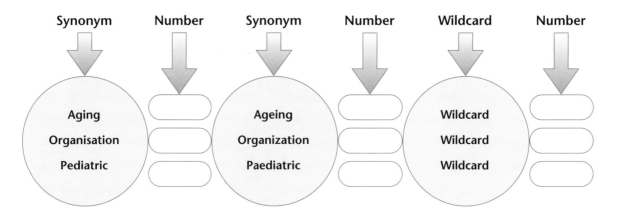

Synonym	Number	Synonym	Number	Wildcard	Number
Aging		Ageing		Wildcard	
Organisation		Organization		Wildcard	
Pediatric		Paediatric		Wildcard	

To continue our pressure sore example:

3. Type in the following words that can also be used to describe pressure sores and mattresses.

    Pressure sore*
    Wound*
    Mattress*

Add these terms to your search strategy by:

4. Combining the terms relating to pressure sores, using the 'OR' Boolean operator.

5. Combining the terms relating to mattresses and beds, using the 'OR' Boolean operator.

6. Combining the two concepts together, using the 'AND' Boolean operator.

Your search will probably look something like this:

9. 7 AND 8
8. 2 OR 6
7. 1 OR 4 OR 5
6. mattress*
5. wound*
4. pressure sore*
3. 1 AND 2
2. beds-and-mattresses
1. pressure-ulcer

7. Compare the results of this search with those of your earlier search (see 'Combining subject/thesaurus terms' above, point 2). What is the difference?

8. Limit this search to clinical trials and reviews.

9. Compare results with those of the earlier limited search (see 'Combining subject/thesaurus terms' above, point 3).

10. Check the results and print out one or two of the most relevant references.

11. Save your search strategy.

This is a basic introduction to building up a search strategy. Sometimes the effects of adding synonyms or using limit features are more dramatic than at other times. Try the same approach with different topic areas to see what happens.

SEARCHING FOR A TOPIC OF INTEREST TO YOU

Think of a topic of interest to you and carry out a literature search on CINAHL for information relating to that topic.

The relevant steps are outlined to get you started.

Step One:
Phrase this idea in a manageable question.

Step Two:
Identify the important components.

Step Three:
Look up relevant subject/thesaurus terms – and perform a search on these subject/thesaurus terms.

Step Four:
Think of alternative synonyms to describe these concepts – and carry out searches on them (remember to use truncation and wildcards where appropriate).

Step Five:
Combine the concepts using Boolean operators.

Step Six:
Apply limits or refine search as necessary.

REPEATING THE SEARCH ON ANOTHER DATABASE

Restricting a search to one database could miss a significant body of evidence.

Repeat either of these searches on a different database available to you. Try and use the most appropriate database for your topic area.

Compare the results you obtained from this database with those obtained from MEDLINE. Was there a large overlap? Were the same key papers retrieved?

Note: If the database you choose uses different software you may have to use different truncation and wildcard symbols. Check the help screens before starting your search.

SUGGESTED ANSWERS

SEARCHING FOR A KNOWN ITEM

1. Find an article by Jenny Popay about qualitative research. Write down the whole reference. Look at the complete record to see how it is laid out and the subject/thesaurus terms (MJ and MN) that have been used to describe the article.

Reference →

Popay J. Rogers A. Williams G. Rationale and standards for the systematic review of qualitative research in health services research. *Qualitative Health Research 8(3): 341–351, 1998.*

Thesaurus terms →

Subject/thesaurus terms:
'health-services-research', 'methods', 'qualitative-studies-methods', 'standards', 'systematic-review-standards'

How to find the answer
Click the author button. Type 'Popay-J' in the search box, click on 'start search'. You can either scroll down the results (if there are a small number) or return to the main search screen and check the 'words anywhere button' and search for the word 'qualitative'. Return to the main search screen and click in the boxes next to the lines you wish to combine and, using the 'AND' Boolean operator, click on the 'combined checked' button to the left of the screen. This will search for papers which mention the word qualitative and the author J Popay.

Click on 'display' to see the records that have been retrieved.

Answers continue

SEARCHING FOR A SUBJECT

Developing a search on the effectiveness of pressure-relieving mattresses on pressure sores.

Using subject/thesaurus terms

1. What is the subject/thesuarus term for pressure sores?

> Pressure-ulcer

How to find the answer
Click on the 'thesaurus' button on the right hand side of the screen. Type the phrase 'pressure sores' into the subject box. Click on 'go to subject'. This will give you a list of potentially relevant subject/thesaurus terms. Select the one you think is most appropriate. Click on the subject/thesaurus term and read the definition to confirm it relates to pressure sores.

2. What is the subject/thesaurus term higher up in the hierarchy (the broader term) for pressure sores?

> Skin-ulcer

How to find the answer
Broader and narrow terms are displayed on the same page as the definition for subject/thesaurus terms.

3. What are the other subject/thesaurus term(s) at the same point in the hierarchy as the subject/thesaurus term for pressure sores?

Leg-ulcer and pyoderma-gangrenosum

How to find the answer
Click on the broader subject/thesaurus term 'skin-ulcer'. This gives you more information about the term and its place in the hierarchy of terms. Narrower and broader terms are also listed. The term 'pressure-ulcer' is a narrower term of 'skin-ulcer', and appears on the same level as 'leg-ulcer' and 'pyoderma-gangrenosum'.

4. Carry out a search for all types of skin ulcers. What function allows you to do this easily?

Explode

How to find the answer
Click on 'skin-ulcer'. Look at the box at the top of the screen. Click on the 'explode subject' button, and then click on the 'explode checked subjects' button. This will search on terms in the subject/thesaurus term hierarchy that you have displayed, in this case all types of skin ulcer.

5. Compare the results of the search for all type of skin ulcers against that for pressure ulcer. What happens when you broaden the search? (Note: This may vary from topic to topic.) What are the implications of this?

A larger number of records are retrieved when the explode function is used. This can be useful if you wish to search a subject comprehensively. However, in this instance, only literature related to pressure sores is wanted. An 'exploded' search in not therefore necessary, as many of the records are likely to be irrelevant because the search includes other types of ulcers.

6. What is the subject/thesaurus term for mattresses?

Beds-and-mattresses

How to find the answer
Click on the 'thesaurus' button on the right hand side of the screen. Type the word 'mattresses' into the subject box. Click on 'go to subject'. This will give you a list of potentially relevant subject/thesaurus terms. Select the one you think is most appropriate. Click on the term and read the definition to confirm it relates to mattresses.

Combining subject/thesaurus terms

1. Combine the subject/thesaurus terms 'pressure-ulcer' and 'beds-and-mattresses'. Ensure you use the 'AND' Boolean operator to obtain the intersection of the two terms.

How to find the answer
Return to the main search screen and click in the boxes next to the lines you wish to combine – 'pressure-ulcer' and 'beds-and-mattresses'. Ensure the 'AND' Boolean operator is selected. Click on the 'combined checked' button to the left of the screen. This will search for papers that mention the terms 'pressure-ulcer' and 'beds-and-mattresses'.

3. Use the limit function to restrict the results to the following document types: 'clinical-trial' and 'review'.

How to find the answer
Return to the main search screen and, on the left hand side of the screen, click in the button 'limit your search'. Scroll down the screen until you see a box entitled 'DT-Document Type'. Use the scroll button of this box to find the limit fields you want, e.g. 'clinical-trial' and 'review'. Hold down the 'Ctrl' key and click the button on the mouse. This will enable you to select more than one limit field at a time. Click on the 'set limits' button in the top right hand corner of the screen.

Now click in the box next to the search line you would like to apply the limit to, and click on the 're-type checked' button on the left of the screen. Click on the 'start search' button next to the search box.

4. Note the other limit features that could have been used.

> Language, publication year

Searching free text

Truncation

1. Type the following terms into CINAHL to see how the truncation function works.

> Asthma*
> Respir*
> Osteo*

Display the articles retrieved. The phrase that you entered will be highlighted in bold. Check to see if articles on subjects you expected were retrieved.

> You should have retrieved articles with a variety of terms including: asthmatics, respiratory, respiration, osteoporosis, osteoarthritis etc.
>
> Note: If you truncate too early you will get irrelevant information. For example, if you were interested in osteoporosis it would be more useful to enter osteop* rather than osteo*.

Wildcards

2. Note the number of articles retrieved for each variation of the spelling. Think of the effect that this would have on the information retrieved if you only searched for one variation of the spelling.

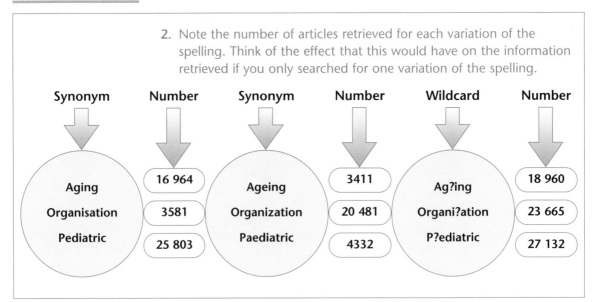

Synonym	Number	Synonym	Number	Wildcard	Number
Aging	16 964	Ageing	3411	Ag?ing	18 960
Organisation	3581	Organization	20 481	Organi?ation	23 665
Pediatric	25 803	Paediatric	4332	P?ediatric	27 132

7. Compare the results of this search with those of your earlier search. What is the difference?

You retrieve more articles and reduce the chance of missing potentially relevant records.

CHAPTER 12

Searching the Internet for healthcare information

Before beginning these exercises, ensure that you know how to access the Internet or NHSnet in your organisation.

Log on to the Internet/NHSnet.

Where appropriate, suggested answers and how to find them are provided on pages 140–146.

ACCESSING A KNOWN WEB SITE

1. Go to the National Institute of Clinical Excellence (NICE) web site at: www.nice.org.uk

2. Practise navigating round the site using the hypertext links.

3. Add the site to your list of favourites.

4. Find the common questions about guidelines. List one of them.

5. Who is responsible for producing guidelines on the 'Induction of Labour'? When were they published?

SEARCHING THE NATIONAL ELECTRONIC LIBRARY FOR HEALTH (NeLH)

(See also Chapter 13.)

1. Go to the NeLH web site at: www.nelh.nhs.uk.

2. Add the site to your favourites.

3. Practise navigating round the site and familiarising yourself with the resources available.

4. List two of the databases that can be accessed via the library. What do they cover?

5. Which resource would you use to find out about recent research?

6. Look at the specialist libraries and editorial resource. Find one that most closely matches your specialty or an area of interest to you. Enter the resource and familiarise yourself with its contents.

7. Find a review of evidence relating to schizophrenia. Write down the reference. Where did you find the review (what source(s) did you use)?

SEARCHING USING A GATEWAY SERVICE

1. Go to the Organising Medical Networked Information (OMNI) gateway service (http://omni.ac.uk/) and add the web site to your bookmark/favourites.

2. Using OMNI find a Health Summit Working Group policy paper on assessing the quality of health information on the Internet. Name the seven criteria the policy paper provides for evaluating web sites.

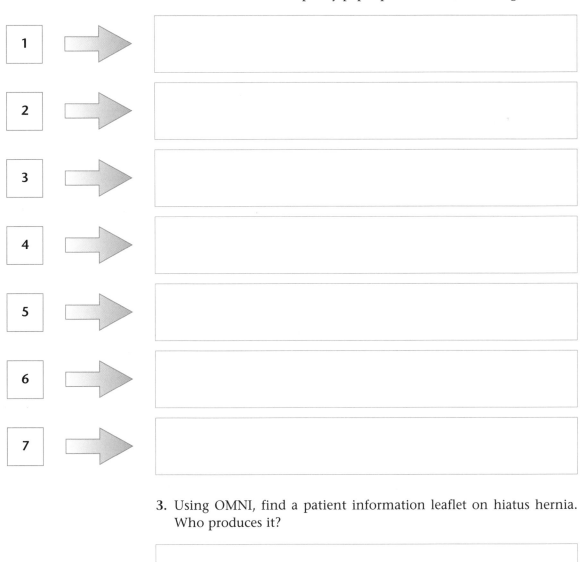

3. Using OMNI, find a patient information leaflet on hiatus hernia. Who produces it?

4. Use OMNI to find the CASP (Critical Appraisal Skills Programme) web site. What critical appraisal checklists are available?

USING A SEARCH ENGINE TO FIND A PARTICULAR SITE

1. Using a search engine of your choice, find the Department of Health web site.

2. What is the web site address?

3. What would you use to find Department of Health publications?

4. Search POINT for a document by Baroness Jay on clinical indicators. What is its title and the briefing series number?

5. Use a search engine of your choice to find the web site of your professional organisation or a professional organisation of interest to you. What is the web address?

SEARCHING FOR INFORMATION ON A PARTICULAR TOPIC

1. Carry out a search on the effectiveness of pressure-relieving mattresses on pressure sores. Try and find good quality evidence. Write down the most relevant reference(s).

2. If you have already completed the similar MEDLINE or CINAHL exercise earlier in the workbook (pages 83–108 or 109–134), compare the method and results.

3. Search for information on a topic of interest to you. Remember to phrase your topic as a question and identify the most important components. It may be useful to search resources in the following order:
   evidence based sources (e.g. knowledge section of NeLH)
   gateway
   professional organisation
   search engine.

4. Practise searching different resources for different questions/topic areas. Remember the Internet is a large, fast changing resource. You may continuously find new and more useful resources and/or find that familiar resources change and are often updated.

SUGGESTED ANSWERS

The answers that follow are suggestions on how to find the information or web site you are interested in. There are numerous ways of searching the Internet; you may easily have chosen a different route to obtain the information you require. Answers are only given where appropriate.

ACCESSING A KNOWN WEB SITE

1. Go to the (NICE) web site at: www.nice.org.uk

2. Practise navigating round the site using the hypertext links.

3. Add the site to your list of favourites.

How to find the answer
Click on the 'favourites' button, click on 'add to favourites'.

---

4. Find the common questions about guidelines. List one of them.

> 1. What is NICE?
> 2. What are Clinical Guidelines?
> 3. Why was NICE asked to develop clinical guidelines? etc.

How to find the answer
Click on 'professional', highlight the 'clinical guidelines' section, then click on 'common questions'. There is a list of questions. You should have selected one of the above.

---

5. Who is responsible for producing guidelines on the 'Induction of Labour'? When were they published?

> Royal College of Obstetricians and Gynaecologists.
> The guidelines were published in June 2001.

How to find the answer
Click on 'clinical guidelines', click on 'completed guidelines and cancer service guidance', scroll down the list until you come to 'Induction of Labour'. Click on link to find out more and access the guideline.

SEARCHING THE NATIONAL ELECTRONIC LIBRARY FOR HEALTH (NeLH)

1. Go to the NeLH web site at: www.nelh.nhs.uk

2. Add the site to your favourites.

3. Practise navigating round the site and familiarising yourself with the resources available.

How to find the answer
Click on the 'favourites' button, click on 'add to favourites'.

4. List two of the databases that can be accessed via the library. What do they cover?

> You could have chosen from the following:
> Cochrane Library 2001/1 – reviews of effectiveness
> Clinical databases
> MEDLINE/PubMed – biomedical literature
> NHS cost and effectiveness reviews
> Research Findings Register – recent research findings of DoH funded projects.

How to find the answer
Go to the NeLH web site at: www.nelh.nhs.uk/ Look at the knowledge section on the left hand side of the screen. Click on the links to find out what resources are available and what they cover.

5. Which resource would you use to find out about recent research?

> Research Findings Register.

How to find the answer
Go to the NeLH web site at: www.nelh.nhs.uk/ Look at the knowledge section on the left hand side of the screen. Click on the links to find out what resources are available and what they cover. The 'Research Findings Register' of DoH funded research is part of this resource.

6. Look at the specialist libraries and editorial resources. Find one that most closely matches your specialty or an area of interest to you. Enter the resource and familiarise yourself with its contents.

> You could have chosen from:
>
> Subjects
>   e.g. Cancer, Health Management
>
> Professions
>   e.g. Nurse, Physiotherapist
>
> Editorial Resources
>   e.g. Telemedicine.

7. Find a review of evidence relating to schizophrenia. Write down the reference. Where did you find the review (what source(s) did you use)?

> Carpenter S, Berk M. Clotiapine for acute psychotic illnesses (Cochrane Review). In: *The Cochrane Library*, Issue 2, 2003. Oxford: Update Software. Located via the Cochrane Library.
>
> Risperidone: efficacy and safety. [Review]. Umbricht D, Kane J M. Schizophrenia Bulletin 1995; 21(4): 593–606. Located via DARE database (NHS Cost and Effectiveness Reviews link).

How to find the answer
Select one of the databases from the knowledge section. Enter the term schizophrenia in the search box. A list of reviews should appear. Select one which seems the most relevant/interesting for your needs. Alternatively enter the term schizophrenia in the pilot search engine box and select a link to an appropriate resource.

SEARCHING USING A GATEWAY SERVICE

1. Go to the Organising Medical Networked Information (OMNI) gateway service (http://omni.ac.uk/) and add the web site to your bookmark/favourites.

2. Using OMNI, find a 'Health Summit Working Group' policy paper on assessing the quality of health information on the Internet. Name the seven criteria the policy paper provides for evaluating web sites.

Criteria for evaluating Internet health information

1. **Credibility:** includes the source, currency, relevance/utility, and editorial review process for the information.
2. **Content:** must be accurate and complete, and an appropriate disclaimer provided.
3. **Disclosure:** includes informing the user of the purpose of the site, as well as any profiling or collection of information associated with using the site.
4. **Links:** evaluated according to selection, architecture, content, and back linkages.
5. **Design:** encompasses accessibility, logical organisation (navigability), and internal search capability.
6. **Interactivity:** includes feedback mechanisms and means for exchange of information among users.
7. **Caveats:** clarification of whether site function is to market products and services or is a primary information content provider.

How to find the answer
Enter OMNI at http://omni.ac.uk In the search box enter a phrase such as quality AND information AND Internet (pick out the most important components of the topic area to help identify terms). Scroll down the list of possible matches to find the correct report. Click on the 'Health Summit Working Group' hypertext link. Click on the 'Health Summit Working Group Policy Paper (html file)' hypertext link. Scan down the document until you reach the box containing the evaluation criteria.

3. Using OMNI, find a patient information leaflet on hiatus hernia. Who produces it?

> Digestive Disorders Foundation.

How to find the answer
Use your bookmark or go to the OMNI web site (http://omni.ac.uk/). Press the return/enter button on your keyboard. Type 'hiatus hernia leaflet' in search field. Scan down the list of possible resources, and click on the hiatus hernia hypertext link. The text of the web page tells you that the Digestive Disorders Foundation produced the leaflet.

4. Use OMNI to find the CASP (Critical Appraisal Skills Programme) web site.

How to find the answer
Enter the gateway at http://omni.ac.uk In the search box, enter CASP. Scroll down the list of results.

5. Locate the CASP critical appraisal checklists. What checklists are available?

> - Randomised controlled trials
> - Economic evaluations
> - Qualitative research studies
> - Systematic reviews of randomised controlled trials
> - Qualitative studies
> - Cohort studies
> - Economic evaluation studies.

How to find the answer
From the 'Public Health Resource Unit' home page, click on 'CASP', select 'Learning Resources', then 'CASP critical appraisal tools'.

USING A SEARCH ENGINE TO FIND A PARTICULAR SITE

1. Using a search engine of your choice, find the Department of Health web site.

2. What is the web site address?

> www.doh.gov.uk/

How to find the answer
Select a search engine. Type 'Department of Health' into the search box. Restrict the search to the UK or add UK to your search.

3. What would you use to find Department of Health publications?

> POINT – Publications Library or
> COIN – Circulars Library (for Executive Letters etc.)

How to find the answer
From the Department of Health web site, click on 'Publications'. Follow the link to the appropriate sources.

4. Search POINT for a document by Baroness Jay on clinical indicators. What is its title and the briefing series number?

> Baroness Jay launches 1996/97 NHS performance (league) tables and announces piloting of 15 clinical indicators. Series: BN11/97.

How to find the answer
Click on 'Publications Library – POINT', Click on 'search Publications only'. Type 'clinical indicators' in the search box. Click on 'search'. Click on file to find title and briefing series number.

SEARCHING FOR INFORMATION ON A PARTICULAR TOPIC

1. Carry out a search on the effectiveness of pressure-relieving mattresses on pressure sores. Try and find good quality evidence. Write down the most relevant reference(s).

> Cullum N, Deeks J, Sheldon TA, Song F, Fletcher AW. Beds, mattresses and cushions for pressure sore prevention and treatment (Cochrane Review). From The Cochrane Library, Issue 2, 2003. Update Software Ltd.
>
> The prevention and treatment of pressure sores: how effective are pressure-relieving interventions and risk assessment for the prevention and treatment of pressure sores? University of York, NHS Centre for Reviews and Dissemination; University of Leeds, Nuffield Institute for Health. Effective Health Care 1995; 2(1): 16 p.

How to find the answer
Use your favourites bookmark button to find the web site of the National Electronic Library for Health. Enter the library. Using the resources in the knowledge section, enter the Cochrane Library and perform a search on pressure sores. Scroll down relevant records. Alternatively try the link for NHS Cost and Effectiveness Reviews. Enter the DARE database. Type in 'pressure sore', choose 'AND', and in second search box type 'mattress'.

Searching the National Electronic Library for Health (NeLH)

Before beginning these exercises, ensure that you know how to access the Internet or NHSnet in your organisation.

Some of the resources available via NeLH are password protected or are available to subscribers only. Contact your library or information service to find out appropriate passwords or services to which they have subscribed.

Where appropriate, suggested answers and how to find them are provided on pages 151–155.

Log on to the Internet/NHSnet and enter the following address:

www.nelh.nhs.uk

FAMILIARISING YOURSELF WITH NeLH

1. Add the site to your favourites.

2. Familiarise yourself with the different sections and resources available.

THE KNOW HOW SECTION

1. Look in the know how section – what does this cover?

2. Find the National Service Framework for Older People.

3. What zone did you find it in?

4. When was it published?

5. What software do you need to view it/print it out?

THE KNOWLEDGE SECTION

1. Look at the knowledge section – what does this cover?

2. List two of the databases that can be accessed via the library. What do they cover?

3. Which resource would you use to find out about recent research?

4. Find a review of evidence relating to schizophrenia. Write down the reference. Where did you find the review (what source(s) did you use)?

SPECIALIST LIBRARIES AND EDITORIAL RESOURCES SECTION

1. Find a specialist library that matches your area of interest. Enter the resource and familiarise yourself with its contents.

SEARCHING FOR INFORMATION ON A PARTICULAR SUBJECT – USING THE PILOT SEARCH ENGINE

The search engine on NeLH searches titles of some of the main items in the 'know how' and 'knowledge' sections.

1. Click on the [more ...] and [help ...] links to find out how it works.

2. Use the search engine to find some information on 'pressure sores'.

3. What resources are you directed to?

4. Did you find as much information as you expected?

EXPANDING YOUR SEARCH – USING THE PILOT SEARCH ENGINE

To improve your chances of finding information, you may need to think of different ways of describing your subject (including alternative spellings or terms/synonyms).

1. Think of different synonyms/spellings to describe 'pressure sores'.

2. Carry out a search using these new terms. (Tip: From the initial pilot search engine box, click on the [search ...] link to find out how to use Boolean operators and other search commands.)

3. How has this affected your results?

EXPANDING YOUR SEARCH – USING SPECIFIC RESOURCES

1. Enter one of the specialist libraries to see what else you can find on 'pressure sores'.

2. If you have already completed a similar MEDLINE/CINAHL/Internet exercise, compare the method and results.

SEARCHING NeLH FOR INFORMATION ON A TOPIC OF YOUR CHOICE

Search for information on a topic of interest to you. The following steps may help you search.

Step One:
Remember to phrase your topic as a question.

Step Two:
Identify the most important components.

Step Three:
Think of alternative synonyms and spellings.

Step Four:
Enter the terms (using Boolean operators) into the pilot search engine.

Step Five:
Follow links through to suggested resources.

Step Six:
Check a relevant specialist library for more information.

SUGGESTED ANSWERS

The answers that follow are suggestions on how to find the information or web site you are interested in. There are alternative ways of searching NeLH; you may easily have chosen a different route to obtain the information you require. Answers are only given where appropriate.

FAMILIARISING YOURSELF WITH NeLH

1. Add the site to your favourites.

How to find the answer
Click on the favourites button, click on 'add to favourites'.

THE KNOW HOW SECTION

1. What does this section cover?

> Frameworks and guidance

How to find the answer
Look in the welcome section and click on the 'where do I look' link.

2. Find the National Service Framework for Older People.

3. What zone did you find it in?

4. When was it published?

5. What software do you need to view/print it?

> **3.** National Service Framework Zone
> **4.** March 2001
> **5.** Adobe Acrobat or view as htm

How to find the answer
Look down the list of resources in the 'know how' section. Click on the National Service Framework Zone. Click on the National Service Framework for Older People.

THE KNOWLEDGE SECTION

1. What does this section cover?

> Searching for evidence

How to find the answer
Look in the welcome section and click on the 'where do I look' link.

2. List two of the databases that can be accessed via the library. What do they cover?

> You should have chosen from the following:
> Cochrane Library 2001/1 – reviews of effectiveness
> NHS Economic Evaluation Database – economic evaluations
> MEDLINE/PubMed – biomedical literature
> Research Findings Register – recent research findings of DoH funded projects
> Reviews of Effectiveness (DARE) – reviews of effectiveness
> DIPEX – via Patient Centred Care Link.

How to find the answer
Look at the knowledge section on the left hand side of the screen. Click on the links to find out what resources are available and what they cover. There are a number of resources that can be used to find evidence in this section. However, not all of them are databases.

3. Which resource would you use to find out about recent research?

> Research Findings Register

How to find the answer
Look at the list of resources in this section. The Research Findings Register – of DoH funded research – is part of this resource.

4. Find a review of evidence relating to schizophrenia. Write down the reference. Where did you find the review (what source(s) did you use)?

Electroconvulsive therapy for schizophrenia. Cochrane Review, Tharyan P and Adams C E. Located via Cochrane Library 2003.

Psychoeducation for schizophrenia. Cochrane Review, Pekkala E and Merinder L. Located via Cochrane Library 2003.

de Olivera I R et al (1996) Risperidone v Haloperidol in the treatment of schizophrenia. Journal of Clinical Pharmacy and Therapeutics 21(5): 349–358. Located via NHS Cost and Effectiveness Reviews.

How to find the answer
Click on Cochrane Library or NHS Cost and Effectiveness Reviews. Enter the resource and perform a search on schizophrenia. Enter the term schizophrenia in the search box. A list of reviews should appear. Select one that seems the most relevant/interesting for your needs. Alternatively go to the pilot search engine, and type schizophrenia. You will be offered a list of possible resources. Select Cochrane and other systematic reviews. Scroll down the page to list relevant reviews. NB: You cannot search the Cochrane Library from this link. You need to exit the pilot search engine and go into the Cochrane Library from the knowledge section.

Answers continue

SEARCHING FOR INFORMATION ON A PARTICULAR SUBJECT – USING THE PILOT SEARCH ENGINE

2. Use the search engine to find some information on 'pressure sores'.

3. What resources are you directed to?

4. Did you find as much information as you expected?

> The answer depends on the term(s) you entered in the pilot search engine. However, if you had used the term 'pressure sores', you would be directed to:
>
> Quality assured summaries (3)
> Cochrane and other systematic reviews (4)
> Original research and study based summaries (3).
> You may have expected to find more information, as there is a wealth of information published on pressure sores. However, the pilot search engine is experimental and only indexes the core content of NeLH. For a complete listing of the resources indexed, check the [help ...] on the pilot search engine.

How to find the answer
Type the term 'pressure sores' into the pilot search engine box. Press 'search'. Scroll down the page to see all the results. Follow links to see appropriate documents. From the NeLH home page check the [more ...] link on the pilot search engine to see how it works.

EXPANDING YOUR SEARCH – USING THE PILOT SEARCH ENGINE

1. Think of different synonyms/spellings to describe pressure sores.

> Pressure ulcer, decubitus ulcer

2. Carry out a search using these new terms. (Tip: Click on the [search tips . . .] link to find out how to use Boolean operators and other search commands.)

3. How has this affected your results?

> More resources have been located. For example, if you typed in 'pressure sore' OR 'pressure ulcer' you may have found:
>
> Guidelines and National Service Frameworks (NSFs) (8)
> Cochrane and other reviews (55)
> Quality assured summaries (6)
> Original research (28).

How to find the answer
Type in the terms 'pressure sore' OR 'pressure ulcer' into the pilot search engine. Press 'search'. The results should appear and you can follow the links to the relevant documents.

EXPANDING YOUR SEARCH – USING SPECIFIC RESOURCES

1. Enter one of the specialist libraries to see what else you can find on pressure sores.

2. If you have already completed a similar MEDLINE/CINAHL/Internet exercise, compare the method and results.

> If you entered the nursing portal the search would locate further items. Entering the terms 'pressure sore' OR 'pressure ulcer' OR 'decubitus' into the search engine would gain more guidelines and Cochrane reviews. Additionally, a search of quality assessed Internet resources produces links to eight relevant items on the NMAP Internet gateway.
>
> In comparison to a search of MEDLINE or CINAHL, a search of NeLH is quite an efficient way of obtaining policy documents and evidence based reviews/summaries. However, it does miss many journal articles. The search engine and interface is much more basic and although you can use Boolean operators and truncation to improve your results there are no thesauri to help. You cannot save your results or strategies.

APPENDICES

Appendix 1. Evaluation tools   159
Appendix 2. Optimal search strategies   165
Appendix 3. Critical appraisal of web sites   167

APPENDIX 1

Evaluation tools

When using information it is important to evaluate its quality and applicability to your particular situation. There is a range of evaluation tools you can use, courses or journal clubs you can attend to develop a thorough understanding of critical appraisal. Three examples of methodological checklists (which appear below) have been developed by the Health Care Practice R&D Unit to assess qualitative and quantitative research studies. Electronic copies of these checklists can also be found at: www.fhsc.salford.ac.uk/hcprdu/assessment.htm

Alternative producers of checklists include the Critical Appraisal Skills Programme in Oxford. Their checklists can be accessed at: www.casp.org.uk Click on 'appraisal checklists'.

EVALUATION TOOL FOR QUALITATIVE STUDIES

Review Area	Key Questions
(1) STUDY OVERVIEW	
Bibliographic Details	Author, title, source (publisher and place of publication), year.
Purpose	What are the aims of the study? If the paper is part of a wider study, what are its aims?
Key Findings	What are the key findings of the study?
Evaluative Summary	What are the strengths and weaknesses of the study and theory, policy and practice implications?
(2) STUDY, SETTING, SAMPLE AND ETHICS	
Phenomena under Study	What is being studied? Is sufficient detail given of the nature of the phenomena under study?

Table continues

Review Area	Key Questions
Context I: Theoretical Framework	What theoretical framework guides or informs the study? In what way is the framework reflected in the way the study was done? How do the authors locate the study within the existing knowledge base?
Context II: Setting	Within what geographical and care setting is the study carried out? What is the rationale for choosing this setting? Is the setting appropriate and/or sufficiently specific for examination of the research question? Is sufficient detail given about the setting? Over what time period is the study conducted?
Context III: Sample (events, persons, times and settings)	How is the sample (events, persons, times and settings) selected? (For example, theoretically informed, purposive, convenience, chosen to explore contrasts.) Is the sample (informants, settings and events) appropriate to the aims of the study? Is the sample appropriate in terms of depth (intensity of data collection – individuals, settings and events) and width across time, settings and events (for example, to capture key persons and events, and to explore the detail of inter-relationships)? What are the key characteristics of the sample (events, persons, times and settings)?
Context IV: Outcomes	What outcome criteria are used in the study? Whose perspectives are addressed (professional, service, user, carer)? Is there sufficient breadth (e.g. contrast of two or more perspectives) and depth (e.g. insight into a single perspective)?
(3) ETHICS	
Ethics	Was Ethical Committee approval obtained? Was informed consent obtained from participants of the study? Have ethical issues been adequately addressed?
(4) DATA COLLECTION, ANALYSIS AND POTENTIAL RESEARCHER BIAS	
Data Collection	What data collection methods are used to obtain and record the data? (For example, provide insight into: data collected, appropriateness and availability for independent analysis.) Is the information collected with sufficient detail and depth to provide insight into the meaning and perceptions of informants? Is the process of fieldwork adequately described? (For example, account of how the data were elicited; type and range of questions; interview guide; length and timing of observation work; note taking.) What role does the researcher adopt within the setting? Is there evidence of reflexivity, that is, providing insight into the relationship between the researcher, setting, data production and analysis?
Data Analysis	How were the data analysed? How adequate is the description of the data analysis? (For example, to allow reproduction; steps taken to guard against selectivity.) Is adequate evidence provided to support the analysis? (For example, includes original/raw data extracts; evidence of iterative analysis; representative evidence presented; efforts to establish validity – searching for negative evidence, use of multiple sources, data triangulation.) Is there reliability/consistency (over researchers, time and settings; checking back with informants over interpretation)? Are the findings interpreted within the context of other studies and theory?
Researcher's Potential Bias	Are the researcher's own position, assumptions and possible biases outlined? (Indicate how those could affect the study, in particular, the analysis and interpretation of the data.)

Review Area	Key Questions
(5) POLICY AND PRACTICE IMPLICATIONS	
Implications	To what setting are the study findings generalisable? (For example, is the setting typical or representative of care settings and in what respects? If the setting is atypical, will this present a stronger or weaker test of the hypothesis?) To what population are the study's findings generalisable? Is the conclusion justified given the conduct of the study? (For example, sampling procedure; measures of outcome used and results achieved.) What are the implications for policy? What are the implications for service practice?
(6) OTHER COMMENTS	
Other Comments	What were the total number of references used in the study? Are there any other noteworthy features of the study? List other study references.
Reviewer	Name of reviewer. Review date.

Evaluation tool last updated: October 2001.

EVALUATION TOOL FOR QUANTITATIVE STUDIES

Review Area	Key Questions
(1) STUDY OVERVIEW	
Bibliographic Details	Author, title, source (publisher and place of publication), year.
Purpose	What are the aims of the study? If the paper is part of a wider study, what are its aims?
Key Findings	What are the key findings of the study?
Evaluative Summary	What are the strengths and weaknesses of the study and theory, policy and practice implications?
(2) STUDY, SETTING, SAMPLE AND ETHICS	
The Study	What type of study is this? What was the intervention? What was the comparison intervention? Is there sufficient detail given of the nature of the intervention and the comparison intervention? What is the relationship of the study to the area of the topic review?
Setting	Within what geographical and care setting was the study carried out?

Table continues

Review Area	Key Questions
Sample	What was the source population? What were the inclusion criteria? What were the exclusion criteria? How was the sample selected? If more than one group of subjects, how many groups were there, and how many people were in each group? How were subjects allocated to the groups? What was the size of the study sample, and of any separate groups? Is the achieved sample size sufficient for the study aims and to warrant the conclusions drawn? Is information provided on loss to follow up? Is the sample appropriate to the aims of the study? What are the key sample characteristics, in relation to the topic area being reviewed?
(3) ETHICS	
Ethics	Was Ethical Committee approval obtained? Was informed consent obtained from participants of the study? Have ethical issues been adequately addressed?
(4) GROUP COMPARABILITY AND OUTCOME MEASUREMENT	
Comparable Groups	If there was more than one group analysed, were the groups comparable before the intervention? In what respects were they comparable and in what were they not? How were important confounding variables controlled (e.g. matching, randomisation, or in the analysis stage)? Was this control adequate to justify the author's conclusions? Were there other important confounding variables controlled for in the study design or analyses and what were they? Did the authors take these into account in their interpretation of the findings?
Outcome Measurement	What were the outcome criteria? What outcome measures were used? Are the measures appropriate, given the outcome criteria? What other (e.g. process, cost) measures are used? Are the measures well validated? Are the measures known to be responsive to change? Whose perspective do the outcome measures address (professional, service, user, carer)? Is there a sufficient breath of perspective? Are the outcome criteria useful/appropriate within routine practice? Are the outcome measures useful/appropriate within routine practice?
Time Scale of Measurement	What was the length of follow-up, and at what time points was outcome measurement made? Is this period of follow-up sufficient to see the desired effects?
(5) POLICY AND PRACTICE IMPLICATIONS	
Implications	To what setting are the study findings generalisable? (For example, is the setting typical or representative of care settings and in what respects?) To what population are the study's findings generalisable? Is the conclusion justified given the conduct of the study? (For example, sampling procedure; measures of outcome used and results achieved.) What are the implications for policy? What are the implications for service practice?
(6) OTHER COMMENTS	
Other Comments	What were the total number of references used in the study? Are there any other noteworthy features of the study? List other study references
Reviewer	Name of reviewer. Review date.

Evaluation tool last updated: October 2001.

EVALUATION TOOL FOR MIXED METHOD STUDIES

Review Area	Key Questions
(1) STUDY OVERVIEW	
Bibliographic Details	Author, title, source (publisher and place of publication), year.
Purpose	What are the aims of this paper? If the paper is part of a wider study, what are its aims?
Key Findings	What are the key findings of the study?
Evaluative Summary	What are the strengths and weaknesses of the study and theory, policy and practice implications?
(2) STUDY, SETTING, SAMPLE AND ETHICS	
The Study	What type of study is this? What is the intervention? What was the comparison intervention? Is there sufficient detail given of the nature of the intervention and the comparison intervention? What is the relationship of the study to the area of the topic review?
Context I: Setting	Within what geographical and care setting is the study carried out? What is the rationale for choosing the setting? Is the setting appropriate and/or sufficiently specific for examination of the research question? Is sufficient detail given about the setting? Over what time period was the study conducted?
Context II: Sample	What was the source population? What were the inclusion criteria? What were the exclusion criteria? How was the sample (events, persons, times and settings) selected? (For example, theoretically informed, purposive, convenience, chosen to explore contrasts.) Is the sample (informants, settings and events) appropriate to the aims of the study? If there was more than one group of subjects, how many groups were there, and how many people were in each group? Is the achieved sample size sufficient for the study aims and to warrant the conclusions drawn? What are the key characteristics of the sample (events, persons, times and settings)?
Context III: Outcome Measurement	What outcome criteria were used in the study? Whose perspectives are addressed (professional, service, user, carer)? Is there sufficient breadth (e.g. contrast of two or more perspectives) and depth (e.g. insight into a single perspective)?
(3) ETHICS	
Ethics	Was Ethical Committee approval obtained? Was informed consent obtained from participants of the study? How have ethical issues been adequately addressed?
(4) GROUP COMPARABILITY	
Comparable Groups	If there was more than one group analysed, were the groups comparable before the intervention? In what respects were they comparable and in what were they not? How were important confounding variables controlled (e.g. matching, randomisation, or in the analysis stage)? Was this control adequate to justify the author's conclusions? Were there other important confounding variables controlled for in the study design or analyses and what were they? Did the authors take these into account in their interpretation of the findings?

Table continues

Review Area	Key Questions
(5) QUALITATIVE DATA COLLECTION AND ANALYSIS	
Data Collection Methods	What data collection methods are used in the study? (Provide insight into: data collected; appropriateness and availability for independent analysis.) Is the process of fieldwork adequately described? (For example, account of how the data were elicited; type and range of questions; interview guide; length and timing of observation work; note taking.)
Data Analysis	How are the data analysed? How adequate is the description of the data analysis? (For example, to allow reproduction; steps taken to guard against selectivity.) Is adequate evidence provided to support the analysis? (For example, includes original/raw data extracts; evidence of iterative analysis; representative evidence presented; efforts to establish validity – searching for negative evidence, use of multiple sources, data triangulation.) Is there reliability/consistency (over researchers, time and settings; checking back with informants over interpretation)? Are the findings interpreted within the context of other studies and theory?
Researcher's Potential Bias	What was the researcher's role? (For example, interviewer, participant observer.) Are the researcher's own position, assumptions and possible biases outlined? (Indicate how these could affect the study, in particular, the analysis and interpretation of the data.)
(6) POLICY AND PRACTICE IMPLICATIONS	
Implications	To what setting are the study findings generalisable? (For example, is the setting typical or representative of care settings and in what respects? If the setting is atypical, will this present a stronger or weaker test of the hypothesis?) To what population are the study's findings generalisable? Is the conclusion justified given the conduct of the study (For example, sampling procedure; measures of outcome used and results achieved.) What are the implications for policy? What are the implications for service practice?
(7) OTHER COMMENTS	
Other Comments	What were the total number of references used in the study? Are there any other noteworthy features of the study? List other study references.
Reviewer	Name of reviewer. Review date.

Evaluation tool last updated: October 2001.

Optimal search strategies

To assist you in identifying specific types of research more effectively, some organisations, such as the NHS Centre for Reviews and Dissemination and the Cochrane Collaboration, have produced search strategies (sometimes referred to as search filters or optimal search strategies).

Optimal search strategies (OSSs) are designed for specific databases and search interfaces. You may require the help of a librarian to translate them to accommodate the software available to you. OSSs are typed into your database in the same way as the search terms identified from your search question, and combined using Boolean operators (as described in Section Two, Chapter 5).

An example of a search strategy developed by the NHS Centre for Reviews and Dissemination to identify reviews and meta-analyses on MEDLINE Ovid looks like this:

1. systematic adj review$.tw.
2. data adj synthesis.tw.
3. published adj studies.ab.
4. data adj extraction.ab.
5. meta-analysis/
6. meta-analysis.ti.
7. comment.pt.
8. letter.pt.
9. editorial.pt.
10. animal/
11. human/
12. 10 not (10 and 11)
13. (YOUR SUBJECT TERMS)
14. 13 not (7 or 8 or 9 or 12)
15. or/1-6
16. 14 and 15.

Other optimal search strategies are available on the following web sites:

❏ Centre for Evidence Based Medicine (2000) *Searching for best evidence in clinical journals*. www.cebm.net/searching.asp

❏ Health Care Practice Research and Development Unit (2000) *An optimal search strategy to identify qualitative research methodologies*. Web site: www.fhsc.salford.ac.uk/hcprdu/

❏ NHS Centre for Reviews and Dissemination (2000) *Search strategies to identify reviews and meta analyses in Medline and Cinahl*. Web site: www.york.ac.uk/inst/crd/search.htm

❏ University of Rochester Medical Center (1999) *Evidence based filters for Ovid Medline*. Web site: www.urmc.rochester.edu/Miner/Educ/Expertsearch.html

❏ University of Rochester Medical Center (1999) *Evidence based filters for Ovid Cinahl*. Web site: www.urmc.rochester.edu/Miner/Educ/ebnfilt.htm

Critical appraisal of web sites

Critical appraisal is important to ensure that information is of good quality and makes sound, evidence based recommendations. This issue is of particular significance in relation to the Internet where information can be made easily available in an unregulated way. Although similar criteria apply to most resources (for example credibility of the author, currency etc.), specific checklists have also been designed for appraising information found on the Internet.

An example is *QUICK: The Quality Information Checklist* (www.quick.org.uk/menu.htm), which provides a set of eight questions, with illustrative examples, to assist in evaluating web sites.

Here are eight ways of checking information on health-related web sites:

❏ Is it clear who has written the information?

❏ Are the aims of the site clear?

❏ Does the site achieve its aims?

❏ Is the site relevant to me?

❏ Can the information be checked?

❏ When was the site produced?

❏ Is the information biased in any way?

❏ Does the site tell you what choices are open to you?

The *Internet Detective* is an interactive tutorial on evaluating the quality of Internet resources, and can be found at: www.sosig.ac.uk/desire/internet-detective.html

Alternatively, additional checklists are included in a bulletin on the topic of the quality assessment of Internet site, available from the Centre for Health Information Quality (1998).

Reference

Centre for Health Information Quality 1998 Quality assessment of Internet sites. Winchester: Centre for Health Information Quality. CHiQ Topic Bulletin Series 2. Web site: www.hfht.org/chiq/download_pdf.htm

Glossary

Applets: Self-contained programs which can be incorporated into web pages to perform a particular function.

Boolean: Boolean operators (or logic) are used for combining search terms. The most common are AND (the intersection of two sets) and OR (the union of two sets).

Browser: A program used to view web pages, e.g. Internet Explorer or Netscape Navigator.

Caching: The storage of copies of web pages previously retrieved so that the speed of future retrievals is enhanced. To ensure that the most current information is presented, the program compares the date of the stored copy with the file at the original location.

Critical appraisal: The process of judging the quality of a study or review and its applicability to practice.

Database: Information stored in a computer system in such a way that it can be easily stored, retrieved and changed.

Directory: A hierarchical and structured database of information which provides a means of searching the Internet.

Email: The sending of text files (in the form of messages) from one computer to another.

Evidence based practice: The process of systematically finding, appraising and using research evidence as a basis for clinical decision-making.

FTP (File Transfer Protocol): A facility for moving files between computers on the Internet.

Gateway service: Quality assessed, access to selected Internet sites in a particular subject area.

Grey literature: Material that can be difficult to track down either because the publisher is unclear, or because the document has been published internally. Also known as report or unpublished literature.

Hypertext links or hyperlinks: The process of linking one web page to another.

Internet: An international 'network of networks' of computers linked together to enable you to communicate with others anywhere in the world.

Java Script or Jscript: A programming language that can be used to enhance the interactivity of web pages.

Limit features: Features provided on some database software interfaces that allow the user to restrict or reduce the search. Common features include age, publication type, publication year and language.

Literature search: The process of finding information, usually from a range of sources.

Mailing lists: Free service to enable discussion of issues and sharing of information via email.

Meta search engine: An Internet search tool that searches a range of search engines and presents the information in a single list.

Newsgroups: Free service to enable discussion of issues and sharing of information via a bulletin board.

Online: A service which is provided electronically via a network, intranet or Internet.

Optimal search strategy/search filter: A published search strategy developed by database 'experts' to retrieve specific types of research study most effectively. The search strategies are designed and tested with particular database and search interfaces in mind.

PDF (Portable Document File): A condensed file which enables large documents to be stored and sent quickly and easily.

Peer review: The assessment of material by a number of 'experts' prior to publication.

Portal: Access to value added services on the Internet such as directories and sites providing links to related web sites.

Precision:	The proportion of relevant information retrieved when undertaking a database search.
Recall:	The amount of available information held by a particular database in relation to your search. Used interchangeably with the term sensitivity.
Search engine:	A searching tool which enables you to find information on a particular subject on the Internet by typing in a word or phrase that describes your area of interest.
Search filter:	See 'Optimal search strategy'.
Search question:	A question which tightly defines the information you are looking for.
Sensitivity:	The amount of available information held by a particular database in relation to your search. Used interchangeably with the term recall.
Systematic review:	A comprehensive review of the evidence in a particular topic area. The review is compiled in a systematic manner, including a comprehensive search of the literature, and critical appraisal and synthesis of the resulting papers.
Thesaurus:	A database 'directory' of preferred search terms, often structured within a hierarchy. Definitions of search terms are often provided.
Vortal:	Access to value added services on the Internet such as directories designed for specific user groups, perhaps defined by subject areas.
WWW (World Wide Web):	The publishing side of the Internet, which allows files placed on the web to be accessed.

INDEX

Notes: Page numbers followed by t indicate tables: page numbers followed by f indicate figures: page numbers followed by p indicate practical exercises

A

ACP Journal Club 21
"address bar" 28
advanced search feature 31, 32f, 33
Aggressive Research Intelligence Facility (ARIF) 20
Allied and Alternative Medicine (AMED) 9t
Alta Vista 33
AMED (Allied and Alternative Medicine) 9t
AOL 34
applets 26, 37
Applied Social Science Index (ASSIA) 9t
Ask Jeeves 34
ASSIA (Applied Social Science Index) 9t

B

Bandolier 17
Best Evidence 21
bias
    qualitative studies 160t
    quantitative studies 164t
"bookmark" 28
books, as sources of information 9, 15
Boolean operators 56
    combining concepts 56–69, 62–64, 69, 93–94p, 98p, 100p
        CINAHL: Ovid interface 111–112p, 119–120p
        CINAHL: SilverPlatter interface 124–125p, 132–133p
        MEDLINE: Ovid interface 85–86p, 93–94p
        MEDLINE: SilverPlatter interface 98–99p, 106–107p
British Library Health Care Information Service 9t
British Medical Journal (BMJ) 21
British Nursing Index 9t
browser 26, 37

C

caching 26, 37
Centre for Evidence Based Medicine 166
Centre for Health Information Quality 168
CINAHL – Cumulative Index to Nursing and Allied Health Literature 9t
CINAHL: Ovid interface 109–121p
    combining concepts 111–112p, 119–120p
    free text 112–114p, 120–121p
    subject headings 110–111p, 117–119p
    truncation 112p, 120p
    wildcards 112–114p, 121p
CINAHL: SilverPlatter interface 122–134p
    combining concepts 124–125p, 132–133p

CINAHL: SilverPlatter interface *contd.*
  free text 125–127p, 133–134p
  subject/thesaurus terms 123–125p,
    130–133p
  truncation 125p, 133p
  wildcards 125–127p, 134p
Cochrane Collaboration
  evidence-based information 18
  optimal search strategies
    165–166
Cochrane Central Register of Controlled
  Trials (CENTRAL) 21
Cochrane Database of Systematic
  Reviews (CDSR) 21
Cochrane Library 10t, 14, 21, 141p,
  152p
  evidence based information 18
Cochrane Methodology Register (CMR)
  21
colleagues, as sources of information
  9
concept method 56–69
Copernic 34
critical appraisal 7, 16, 35–36, 36,
    39, 76
  evaluation tools 159–164
  literature searching (*see* literature
    searching)
  web sites 167–168
Critical Appraisal Skills Programme
  159
CSP Databases 10t

D

Database of Abstracts of Reviews of
  Effects (DARE) 21, 152p
databases 9–11, 9t–10t. *see also*
    individual databases
  advantages/disadvantages 9t–10t
  evidence based information 21
  literature searching 56–69
  optimal search strategies 21,
    165–166
  as sources of information 14
data collection/analysis
  qualitative studies 160t
  quantitative studies 164t
DH-Data 10t
Diagnostic Strategies for Common
  Medical Problems 21

digests 17
DIPEX 152p
directory 26, 34, 37

E

Effective Health Care (EHC) 17
Effectiveness Matters 17
electronic databases. *see* databases
Email 26, 37
Embase 10t, 14
ethics
  qualitative studies 160t
  quantitative studies 162t,
    163t
evaluation tools 159–164
evidence based information
  advantages 16, 22, 24
  sources 16–24
    databases 21
    Internet 16–17
    journals/newsletters 17–18
    optimal search strategies (OSSs)
      163–164
    organisations 18
    reports 19–20
Evidence Based Medicine 17
Evidence Based Mental Health 17
Evidence Based Midwifery 17
Evidence Based Nursing 17
Excite 33

F

"favourites button" 28
File Transfer Protocol (FTP) 26, 37
find function 29
free text (*see also* synonyms,
    identification)
  CINAHL: Ovid interface
    112–114p, 120–121p
  CINAHL: SilverPlatter interface
    125–127p, 133–134p
  MEDLINE: Ovid interface 86p,
    94–95p
  MEDLINE: SilverPlatter interface
    99–101p, 107–108p
FTP (File Transfer Protocol) 26,
  37

G

gateway service 26, 34, 37,
    137–138p, 143–144p
Google 34
"grey" literature
    organisations 18
    as source of information 12, 19–20

H

*Health Care Practice Research and
    Development Unit* 159, 166
    web page (example) 28f–29f
Health Evidence Bulletins 17
help menu 73
"history button" 29
"home button" 28
Hot Bot 33
hypertext links 26, 29, 37

I

indexes, as sources of information
    9–11, 15
Index Medicus 10t
information
    critical appraisal 35
    evaluation tools 159–164
    evidence based (*see* evidence based
        information)
    sources 7–15
        advantages/disadvantages 9t–10t
        Internet (*see* Internet)
information retrieval. *see* literature
        searching
Internet 25–39, 76
    databases (*see* databases)
    definition 11, 25, 27, 37
    as information source
        advantages/disadvantages 11,
            14, 15
        evidence based information
            16–17
    literature searching 31–39,
        135–146p
        advantages/disadvantages 14
        Boolean operators (*see* Boolean
            operators)
        evaluation criteria 143p

expanding searches 73
    limiting searches 48–49, 73
    refining searches 64–65, 73
    text word searching 60–61
    tips 72–73
    search engines (*see* search engines
        (Internet))
    terminology 26–30
    web browsers 27–29, 28f, 30 (*see
        also* individual browsers)
    web site addresses (*see also*
        individual Internet sites)
        critical appraisal 167–168
        structure 29–30
Internet Detective 82p, 167
Internet Explorer 26, 27–28
*Irish Clearing House on Health
    Outcomes (ICHHO)* 18
Ixquick 34

J

Java Script 27, 37
Joseph Rowntree Foundation 18
*Journal of the American Medical
    Association (JAMA)* 21
journals. *see also* individual journal
    titles
    evidence based information 17–18,
        23
    peer reviewed 23
    as source of information 11, 15
    subject-specific 17
Jscript 27, 37

K

keywords, allocation 11

L

libraries, as source of information 15
literature searching 43–55. *see also
    under* CINAHL; MEDLINE
    attitudes to 3, 70–71
    constraints 45
    critical appraisal 7, 16, 35–36, 39, 76
        evaluation tools 159–164
        web sites 167–168

literature searching *contd.*
  definition 43
  evaluation tools 159–164
  information sources
    databases (*see* databases)
    identification 45
  Internet (*see* Internet)
  optimal search strategies 21,
    165–166
  search questions 45, 46–55, 56
    clarification 50, 54, 75
    combining concepts 62–64, 69,
      85–86p, 98–99p, 111–112p
      (*see also* Boolean operators)
    concept identification/
      description 48, 53, 60–61
  stages 56–69
  subject/thesaurus terms 97–98p,
    104–106p, 110–111p,
    123–125p, 130–133p
literature, "unpublished", as source
  of information 12
location bar 28
Lycos 33

M

mailing lists 27, 37
MEDLINE 9, 10t, 14, 57f, 152p
MEDLINE: Ovid interface 83–95p
  combining terms 85–86p, 93–94p
  free text 86p, 94–95p
  MESH/subject headings 84–85p,
    91–93p
  strategies 165
  truncation 86p, 94p
  wildcards 86–88p, 95p
MEDLINE: SilverPlatter interface
    96–108p
  combining terms 98–99p,
    106–107p
  free text 99–101p, 107–108p
  truncation 99p, 107p
  using subject/thesaurus terms
    97–98p, 104–106p
  wildcards 99–101p, 108p
MESH hierarchy 58f, 64, 69, 84–85p,
    91–93p
MetaCrawler 34
meta search engines 34
MSN 33

N

*National Coordinating Centre for
  Health Technology Assessment
  (NCCHTA)* 20
National Electronic Library for
  Health 7, 21, 34, 82p
  searches 141–142p, 147–155p,
    154–155p
    Pilot Search Engine 149–150p,
      154p
*National Institute for Clinical
  Excellence (NICE)* 19, 23
Netscape Navigator 27–28
*New England Journal of Medicine
  (NEJM)* 21
newsgroups 27, 38
newsletters, evidence based
  information 17–18, 23
*NHS Centre for Reviews and
  Dissemination (CRD)* 19, 20,
    23, 24, 166
  optimal search strategies
    165–166
NHS Direct Online 34
NHS Economic Evaluation
  Database 152p
NMAP 34

O

OMNI 34
optimal search strategies (OSSs) 21,
    165–166
organisations, professional
  evidence based information
    18–19, 19, 20, 23, 24
  as source of information 11, 14, 15
Ovid interface. *see* CINAHL: Ovid
    interface; MEDLINE: Ovid
    interface

P

PDF (Portable Document File) 27, 38
phrasing
  definition 31
  search questions (*see* literature
    searching)

PICO method 49–50, 51, 55
policy implications
    qualitative studies 161t
    quantitative studies 160t, 164t
portals 27, 34
Practical exercises
    CINAHL: Ovid interface 109–121p
    CINAHL: SilverPlatter interface
        122–134p
    MEDLINE: Ovid interface 83–95p
    MEDLINE: SilverPlatter interface
        96–108p
"print button" 29
professional organisations
    evidence based information
        18–19, 20, 23, 24
    as source of information 11, 14, 15
"Protocols" 29
Psychlit 10t
PsycInfo (Psychlit) 10t
PubMed 82

Q

qualitative studies, evaluation tools
    159t–161t
Quality Information Checklist (QUICK)
    35, 167
quantitative studies, evaluation tools
    161t–164t, 162
questions, search. see literature
    searching
QUICK (Quality Information Checklist)
    35, 167

R

ranking 31
"refresh button" 28
reports
    evidence based information 19–20
    as source of information 12
Research Findings Register 141p, 152p

S

sampling
    qualitative studies 160t
    quantitative studies 162t, 163t

"search button" 28
search engines (Internet) 27, 31–34,
    32f, 138p, 145p. see also
    individual search engines
    definition 27, 38
    simple/advanced feature 32f
search filters 21
search questions. see literature
    searching
SilverPlatter interface. see CINAHL:
    SilverPlatter interface;
    MEDLINE: SilverPlatter
    interface
"Site address" 29
Sociofile 10t
"stop button" 28
subject terms 110–111p
    CINAHL: SilverPlatter interface
        123–125p, 130–133p
    MEDLINE: SilverPlatter interface
        97–98p, 104–106p
synonyms, identification 60–61, 68
systematic reviews 43–44

T

text word searching 60–61
theoretical framework, qualitative
    studies 160t
thesaurus terms 110–111p
    CINAHL: SilverPlatter interface
        123–125p, 130–133p
    MEDLINE: SilverPlatter interface
        97–98p, 104–106p
Tonic 82p
TRIP Database 21
truncation 61, 62, 68, 86p, 99p,
    112p, 125p
    CINAHL: Ovid interface 112p,
        120p
    CINAHL: SilverPlatter interface
        125p, 133p
    MEDLINE: Ovid interface 86p, 94p
    MEDLINE: SilverPlatter interface
        99p, 107p

U

University of Rochester Medical
    Center 166

"unpublished" literature, as source of information 12
URL (Uniform Resource Locator) 28

V

Venn diagrams 63–64, 69
Virtual Training Suite 82p
vortals 27, 35

W

web browsers 27–29, 28f, 30
web site addresses. *see* Internet
WebSPIRS. *see* CINAHL: SilverPlatter interface; MEDLINE: SilverPlatter interface

wildcards 61–62, 68, 86–88p, 99p, 112–114p, 125–127p
    CINAHL: Ovid interface 112–114p, 121p
    CINAHL: SilverPlatter interface 125–127p, 134p
    MEDLINE: Ovid interface 86–88p, 95p
    MEDLINE: SilverPlatter interface 99–101p, 108p
WinSPIRS. *see* CINAHL: SilverPlatter interface; MEDLINE: SilverPlatter interface
WWW (World Wide Web). *see* Internet

Y

Yahoo 34